Teachings on Healing
From a Spiritual Perspective

Teachings on Healing
From a Spiritual Perspective

THIRD EDITION

Gabriel of Urantia
& Niánn Emerson Chase

Global Community Communications Publishing

Tubac / Tumacácori, Arizona, USA

First Edition published 2002

ISBN 978-0-9822423-0-8

Global Community Communications Publishing
P.O. Box 4910, Tubac, Arizona 85646 USA
(520) 603-9932
e-mail: info@GlobalCommunityCommunicationsPublishing.org
www.GlobalCommunityCommunicationsPublishing.org

COVER ART: *Life Pattern* is an original art piece (6' x 4') in mixed medium of acrylic and art glass on board by Ausmaminae, a CosmoArtist from Global Community Communications Alliance in Arizona, USA. The Universe Mother Spirit, as part of the sevenfold channel of the river of life, lovingly stirs the living waters as she vitalizes the life patterns upon each evolving world. "Life flows from the Father, through the Son, and by the Spirit." (*The URANTIA Book*, p. 404) The Divine Mother's loving presence serves as a constant reminder to us all of the revitalizing and renewing energies of birth and healing ever-available to all God's children throughout eternity. For more information or to purchase a variety of CosmoArt, go to the Web site at www.cosmoart.org, contact via e-mail info@cosmoart.org, or call (520) 398-9409.

Contents

Introduction

The teachings presented in this book are a compilation of years of personal growth, experiences, and study in the lives of the authors, Gabriel of Urantia and Niánn Emerson Chase, dedicated spiritual leaders and teachers.

Four of the teachings—"Integrated, Wholistic Healing: Eco-Systems, Social-Systems, and Person-Systems," "Healing Through Feeling," "Healing Through Kneeling," and "Rendezvousing with the Rainbow"—were previously published in the quarterly periodical the *Alternative Voice*. Half of the teachings in this compilation are jointly presented by Niánn Emerson Chase and Gabriel of Urantia—except where noted otherwise. "The Quantum World and The Physics of Healing" by Gabriel of Urantia was first published in the bi-monthly magazine *Innerchange* (June/July 2006).

If you come across some unfamiliar terms in this book, please check the abbreviated glossary, as the terms are probably defined there. All of the glossary terms are terms introduced by epochal revelation.

Throughout this book, there are many references to Global Community Communications Alliance, the nonprofit, spiritual educational organization that Gabriel and Niánn co-founded in 1989, presently based in Arizona, USA. Often Global Community Communications Alliance is also referred to as *Divine Administration* or the *First Planetary Sacred Home*.

For more information about Global Community Communications Alliance and the other outreach ministries of Gabriel of Urantia and Niánn Emerson Chase, please refer to the back of this book or visit:

www.GlobalCommunityCommunicationsAlliance.org.

Integrated, Wholistic Healing: Eco-Systems, Social-Systems, and Person-Systems

by Niánn Emerson Chase

Recently I explained to my primary healthcare physician how I saw our relationship:

You are my physician, my only doctor at this time. This is my choice. I trust you over any other doctor when it comes to my personal health, but I also "tune in" to my own body and what I intuit is best for me. I see our doctor-patient relationship as a collaboration, a team effort, for it is not really up to you to solve my health problems, but up to me. You're there to assist me, and I value your experience, your knowledge, your wisdom, and your godliness. I know that you have my highest good in mind when you act as my physician, and I trust you. I won't always agree with your opinions or suggestions, but I will always consider them.

In spite of my physical aging process and increased limitations, I think I am healthier than I have ever been in my entire life. My overall health just keeps getting better because my psychospiritual health just keeps getting better. I feel strong and more balanced physically, emotionally, intellectually, and spiritually than ever before. Though I no longer can do certain things physically that I could do fifteen or twenty years ago, I can do many other things that I couldn't do two decades ago, mostly on the intellectual and psychospiritual levels.

You are my dear beloved physician, friend, and fellow minister. You have been an integral part of my ongoing improving overall health and well-being. Thank you, my doctor friend, for your dedicated love, humility, flexibility, openness, and collaboration in this continuing process of remaining healthy. I feel blessed by God to have you by my side in a physician's role, and I hope that all of your other patients have similar sentiments.

I realize that most patients do not feel that way about their doctors, at least in this country. But there have always been some exceptional doctors in every generation, doctors who are in the ministry of caring for the well-being of others rather than in the business of healthcare. My primary-care doctor is one of those exceptional people, and so are others from the past as well as in the present. These exceptional ones are of various races, religions, and nationalities and include both men and women. I realize that healthcare should involve an integration of considering the whole person, which includes the entire physical body-system, as well as the emotional, mental, and spirit systems of the individual.

Interestingly, as an avid student and teacher of the concepts found in *The URANTIA Book*, I have noted that when referring to the health of a person, this wonderful spiritually-based text associates “health” with the body, mind, and soul. Health is linked with sensible living habits, happiness, mental clarity, emotional stability, and an awareness of spiritual reality.

> Health, sanity/mental efficiency, and happiness are integrations of truth, beauty, and goodness as they are blended in human experiences. Such levels of efficient/balanced living come about through the unification of the energy/physical systems, idea/mind systems, and spirit systems. (See pages 43 and 1097 of *The URANTIA Book*)

Rather than compartmentalizing human beings into separate parts to be “treated” by specialists, exceptional healthcare givers/ministers have more of a "wholistic" perspective when interacting with those they are attempting to aid in becoming healthier, by integrating and unifying and blending parts rather than separating them out.

The more progressive healthcare providers, scientists, sociologists, educators, theologians, and statespersons (rather than mere politicians) realize that in treating "sick" environments, societies, and persons you have to look at the entire eco-systems, social-systems, and person-systems. The declining health of Mother Earth matches and is interlinked with the declining health of our modern societies and individual citizens.

In my own struggles to maintain good health and well-being, I have discovered that my own life-support systems seem to match the Earth's and its peoples. As the lungs of the Earth are being debilitated by the massive destruction of rain forests, my lungs feel compromised too. As the Earth's waterways are being poisoned and depleted, so does my circulatory system feel sluggish and inefficient. As people's hearts are broken and their spirits diminished by a consumer-driven, mechanistic social system, so my heart feels fragile with my grieving over the cold-hearted state of the dominant culture.

I think that poor health—whether in a person or in our natural world or in a society—is a result of being out of divine pattern. Divine pattern involves integrative systems that all coordinate to reflect the truth, beauty, and goodness of God, and, frankly, a vast majority of religious endeavors and institutions on this world are not healthy at all, regardless of their religious rhetoric. They are very sick and have been out of divine pattern for many thousands of years.

Tens of thousands of years ago the ancient Sethite priesthood was comprised of "high-minded and noble teachers of health and religion" who were "true educators" and not at all like most of the "debased" and "commercialized" religious teachers and healthcare providers of today (*The URANTIA Book*, p. 850). Socrates and his successors, Plato and Aristotle, taught that goodness was the health of the soul (*The URANTIA Book*, p. 1079). Today, only a few healthcare professionals—who are caught in the ocean of a grasping, greedy medical industrial complex—realize the truth that people's health is tied up with the state of their souls.

The work that I am involved in, which encompasses every aspect of my life, integrates all life experiences into a whole. My own healing process has been one of becoming uncompartmentalized and more unified within my whole being. The Soulistic Medical Institute, which is a facet of my work, has another way of looking at "health." It has redefined health in its outreach ministries of providing healthcare, just as I have had to continually redefine what good health is for me as I unfold into my God-given personality circuitry and grow psychospiritually.

In my own health-maintenance process I rarely use "health professionals" and medicines because I don't need to. Though very full with meaningful work and many responsibilities, my lifestyle is less strenuous and rushed than twenty years ago. I eat organically-grown foods from our Avalon Gardens; drink clean, chemical-free water from our private wells; exercise by daily walking and hiking in beautiful natural places; and use eco-friendly common products for home, lawn, and personal care. In not using toxic foods and products, I don't poison myself or my natural environment. And I feel good mentally in taking responsibility for caring for my physical health and for my natural environment.

Even more importantly, in taking responsibility for my own health is the overseeing of my psychospiritual welfare. I spend time reading and expanding intellectually. I interact closely with fellow kindred spirits and good friends in an intentional-community setting. And I laugh—at myself and at the many silly situations in life on this world.

Some healthcare professionals realize that the use of humor in the treatment of diseases and health promotion is integral in healing. "Humor serves a valuable purpose both as a health insurance and as a liberator of emotional pressure, thus preventing injurious nervous tension and overserious contemplation." (*The URANTIA Book*, p. 549)

In the maintenance of my own health, I rest, contemplate, meditate, reflect, pray, and worship. I have come to fully embrace the truth that an understanding at some level of spiritual reality can contribute to the enjoyment of abundant health and to the cure of numerous mental, emotional, and nervous ailments.

> Even the physical problems of bodily health and efficiency are best solved when they are viewed from the religious standpoint of our Master's [Jesus'] teaching: That the body and mind of mortals are the dwelling place of the gift of the Gods, the Spirit of God becoming the spirit of man and woman. The mind of men and women becomes the mediator between material things and spiritual realities. (*The URANTIA Book*, p. 1779)

> The joy of the outpoured spirit, when it is consciously experienced in human life, is a tonic for health, a stimulus for mind, and an unfailing energy for the soul. (*The URANTIA Book*, p. 2065)

Cellular biologist Dr. Bruce Lipton emphasizes that our beliefs can change how our genes will respond. He states: "The new science has everything to do with your beliefs." Though Dr. Lipton calls this awareness "new science," the fact that energy follows thought has been known in the circles of genuine religious persons for thousands of years.

Now with the new science a small number of progressive scientists and healthcare professionals are beginning to understand the power of thought and how energy in body systems is affected by the state of mind in individuals. With thinking and attitudes that are founded on truth, beauty, and goodness, there is a greater probability for healing. Beliefs and perspectives that are negative, resentful, self-centered, and fear-based can cause poor health. In addition, the beliefs and energy fields of other people around an individual can affect how healthy or unhealthy that individual will be.

The teachings presented in this book are based upon common sense combined with spiritual insights in the overall approach to healing. They reflect the need for a wholistic treatment of a person with an illness or disease, addressing body, mind, and soul. The concepts presented in these teaching are founded on the premise of wholehearted participation on the part of the patient, in order for true healing to occur, always and ever recognizing the hand of God in our lives and the importance of doing His will first and foremost in order to flow within the harmony of the grand universe.

Vignettes: Healing Through Feeling

by Niánn Emerson Chase

Five years before his death at age sixty-seven, my father was diagnosed with cancer. He had four years of a full, active life, and then he became too pain-ridden and debilitated in his last year before graduating from this world. From my perspective, my beloved and dignified father, Leland Dean Chase, had a quality life up to the very end in spite of the physical deterioration of his body.

I observed my father go through much healing and growth in his last five years. Though my father was always a compassionate, gentle man, his "edges" became softer and rounder. The virtues he was known for—moral strength and spiritual stability—just became stronger and more crystal clear as he opened himself to expanding his understanding of life and changing his thinking about certain things. His acceptance of the differences in some of his family members deepened, and his great love for us became even greater.

I too experienced much healing during the time my dad was physically dying but, paradoxically, really healing. I became comforted and at peace with the situation my father was going through as I observed his own psychospiritual growth unfold. Interestingly, my own inner healing and growth was enhanced by his.

Though always good, our relationship got better because we were aware of the shortness of time he had on this world. We both grew in our appreciation of each other; we flowed more naturally with each other, outgrowing the inappropriate expectations we had clung to for so many years. We learned to just enjoy the other's presence. We both grew in our gratitude for life and for the daily gifts that life bestows upon all of us.

Though cancer eventually got my father's body, it did not get him. He lives on in the memories of all of those who loved him, and I know he lives on—in another body (a morontia body), on another world (a mansion world). I look forward to seeing him again.

I lost two other close, life-long friends to the plague of cancer. When diagnosed with this terrible disease, both were given by their doctors six months at the most, regardless of any treatment they would take. (Sometimes I think that six months is the catch-all time given for patients when there is supposedly no hope.) Both chose not to travel the arduous road of the typical methods of treatment found in the medical field—surgery, chemotherapy, and radiation—and selected more natural methods that were considered alternative at the time.

Both had a strong, dynamic faith in the loving presence of God in their lives, and both believed that they could be healed miraculously. Many people, including me, prayed for their physical survival and victory over cancer. As with my father, I saw much healing happen for each one of these dear people, though one passed on almost six months to the day after his diagnosis. The other one, in defiance of her doctors' dire prognosis, lived two years beyond the predicted six months!

I have to say honestly that both of these individuals were happier and more at peace in their last months and years than I had ever seen before their diagnosis of cancer. Naturally, they initially struggled with the knowledge of having a life-threatening illness, but they both shifted in their perceptions of their reality as they succumbed to resting in their Creator's hands.

I think that as they experienced the fragility of their physical, temporal existence, an awareness of their other-than-physical, eternal realness became more prominent in their consciousness—thus, their increased happiness and healing as they lived fully in the moment and looked forward to a future full of new experiences and discoveries. I think they looked at their inevitable deaths as crossing a bridge into an even more exciting adventure.

Another friend of mine, at seventeen years of age, was diagnosed with rheumatoid arthritis (by more than one doctor) and told that by the time she was twenty-five she would be in a wheel chair for the rest of her life. An active athlete, this teenager informed the doctors that she would show them how wrong they were when *she walked* into their office eight years later. And she did. I first met her when she was in her early thirties, still an athlete on her feet. Two decades later, at 56 she has had a family, changed her career twice, plays tennis (on her feet), rides mountain bikes, and backpacks into wilderness areas. There's no wheel chair sitting around her place.

When I asked her why this disease did not "get" her, she said, "Because I did not accept the diagnosis. I would not let my mind stay focused on the possibility of me having this disease. I pretty much ignored my pain and continued being just as active physically as I always had been. I did not buy into the gig the doctors offered me, and therefore it was not a part of my reality."

My friend's mind certainly seemed to wipe out her physical illness. It has been said that energy follows thought, and this most certainly seems to be the case here.

In reflecting upon my own life, I recall times when I have felt "dis-eased." At about age five I had begun experiencing a vague sense of "mission," which continued to unfold, and in my pubescent years the "knowing" that I had a destiny in helping to make the world better suddenly became more apparent and continued to intensify throughout my teen years. In my childhood I had colds, measles, chicken pox, and so on, but I did not feel dis-eased with those childhood ailments.

When I was around twelve I became very weak and listless. I started chewing the skin of my fingers as if I was frustrated or haunted by something, but what that something was I could not identify. The various medical tests showed no physiological cause for these symptoms except for a slight case of anemia, and when my physician (and family friend) asked me if there was anything in my life that was bothering or upsetting me, I could think of nothing out of the ordinary.

That was the problem—my life seemed too ordinary; nothing extraordinary was happening! My whole being was wanting something more than I had, and I had a very good life—with devoted and loving parents and siblings, as well as fun-loving extended family and friends; living on an Indian reservation with clean, open spaces to roam (which I loved doing); having an active, intellectual life of avid reading; and living a dynamic religious faith with an interesting combination of Native American spirituality and Christianity. What in Heaven's name was wrong with me?

In actuality, nothing was really wrong and almost everything in my life was right except that I yearned for something more—something very elusive, something I could not name. And that yearning (for something that I could not do anything about) is what I was not at ease with, thus the "dis-ease." After several months of suffering this minor melancholy, I suddenly made a shift, becoming lively and enthusiastic again, and the skin on my fingers began to heal since I no longer chewed on them.

Two thousand years ago Jesus was asked by one of His apostles, "Why are some persons so much more happy and contented than others? Is contentment a matter of religious experience?" In His lengthy answer, Jesus included this:

> . . . [S]ome persons are naturally more happy than others. Much, very much, depends upon the willingness of an individual to be led and directed by the Father's spirit which lives within him [or her]. (*The URANTIA Book*, p. 1674)

I think that in my pre-teen prayers for healing what was ailing me, I received help from the Threefold Spirit within. I believe that the Holy Spirit of the Universe Mother Spirit kept nurturing me and reinforcing the comfort and messages that the Spirit of Truth was giving me. Because I was sincere in my desire to move out of my dis-ease, my heart and mind were open and receptive, and thus the Fragment of the Father (Spirit of God) was able to help me change my mind, adjust my thoughts of dissatisfaction and obsessive yearning. In other words, I was able to shift into gratitude and the attitude of "be here now," be in the eternal present.

Though I do think that innate within all humans is the desire to always reach for something higher, something even more divine, we also have to recognize the times when we are where God wants us, and we must be content in our moments, and that is what, at age twelve, I began to learn to manifest.

In hindsight, decades later, I understand that in those tender and sensitive years of puberty when I was shifting into an adult mind and body, at a cellular level my heart was remembering other realities closer to divine pattern that I had experienced on another world in another universe, and I was grieving the loss of that existence and experiencing the frustration of living in a culture of lower consciousness.

Years later, when I was a sophomore in college I went through another dis-ease episode, suffering from similar symptoms of my previous, pubescent melancholy. Again, nothing was found in all of the medical tests I went through to explain my extreme lack of energy, dizzy spells, and horrible rashes running up my legs and back. Again, there seemed to be nothing untoward in my life happening that would be the cause of this sudden demise in vibrancy. But this time I was more aware of the cause of my uneasiness, and I recall having long, emotional phone conversations with my father about my inner struggle. Though he was at a loss in how to help me solve my psychological and spiritual turmoil, my father was always available when I called out for help. He listened to me, prayed with me, and simply loved me.

I think that my earthly father's loving, parental presence helped me to open up more to my heavenly Father's guiding, healing presence. I think that my human father shared his own particles of stability and strength with me, thus aiding me as I went through the healing process with my First Father.

Unlike my human father, who was a first-light soul, I, who am a starseed, have layers of past-life experiences, with layers of codes imbedded at a cellular level that I must acknowledge and eventually decipher. As an undergraduate university student I again was faced with memories of saner and safer worlds more evolved than this one. I again felt the strong sense of responsibility for contributing to the advancement of this world, and I experienced frustration at being so stuck in so many limitations and so alone in my realizations.

I again received the ministry of living spiritual forces and, after three months, my physical symptoms of dis-ease abated. I was comforted and felt more strongly committed to my sense of service to the world. Again I felt reassured that I was, in that moment in time and space, where I was meant to be, finishing my work in school.

Though, since college, I have gone through many minor instances of dis-ease with my circumstances, I consider only two other episodes that seemed huge, and discussion of those are for another time. Obviously I am still here, and those episodes of illness did not get me—either physically or psychospiritually. In fact, as a result of those episodes, I have had great *healing*. I feel healthier than I ever have—physically, emotionally, intellectually, and spiritually. I no longer have a twenty-year-old body, or a thirty-, or even a forty-year-old body, but it has slowed to the tempo of the universe, to the tempo of the cosmologic vibration pattern that is being reestablished on this world, and so my heart and cells continue to open up to the code of divine pattern. (See Paper 216 of *The Cosmic Family, Volume I* for further discussion of "cosmologic vibration pattern.")

I think that well-being has to do with *relationship*—relationship with our Creator, with living spiritual forces and personalities, with other humans, with our place in the universe and on this world. Well-being has to do with our perceptions of reality, of ourselves, of others.

French author Marcel Proust, whose writing explores the influence of past experience on present reality, once stated, "The real voyage of discovery consists not in seeking new lands but in seeing with new eyes." I think that true healing has to do with seeing with new eyes, spiritized eyes.

Healing by Kneeling
. . . with a Little Help from Our Friends

by Gabriel of Urantia

Many articles and books have been written on the subject of healing, so I would like to be as precise as possible without beating around the holy bush. First of all, if you look at any of the New Age periodicals and see all of the healers listed, you would think that no one should be sick at all! The fact is, however, people do die of all kinds of diseases and live physically painful lives even though all these healers are out there making all kinds of fantastic claims. There's always a new method and a larger price to pay to someone who claims to have the answers to your illness. The pharmaceutical industry has the drug for every ailment, and the New Age healers have the metaphysical new touch to alleviate your every pain.

The fact is that supernatural healings do happen. I have experienced this in the past, in my own life as well as in the lives of others, with healers who truly have a mandate from God to heal, like the deceased Katherine Coleman. She was the first to tell you that it was the power of God that healed, not her. I also believe that God does use individuals to help in the healing process.

For thousands of years, Chinese acupuncture as well as sound and music therapy, healing mineral waters, crystal energy, and herbology have worked in many ailments of the body. Even massage has worked to alleviate muscle pains and circulation problems. But rather than go on and list a thousand and one others, there is a spiritual truth that needs to be looked at for any healing to take place and an understanding that some healings will not completely take place due to no spiritual fault of the individual.

The secret of the mystery of illness and healing has to do with *destiny*. First of all, you cannot understand destiny unless you understand that there is a God who created you, who knows you, and who has a destiny specifically for you to meet in every area of your life. Your career, life partner, and significant others are some of those essentials that God foreordains for every individual. The problem is that when billions of individuals are making wrong choices in so many significant areas of their own lives, this affects your life too.

This principle is understood to some degree by those on a spiritual path, but not to the degree necessary, or else we would have a world of wholeness and fulfillment. In order to properly teach the concept of meeting one's destiny, it would truly take a master in a spiritual school like those that are on some higher worlds of time and space. Here in Arizona, these teachings are offered in Global Community Communications Schools, concept upon concept and precept upon precept.

In relation to the concept of destiny, millions of individuals become ill with certain symptoms, like diabetes. Many of the Native Americans, who were nomadic hunters and gatherers, suffer from diabetes because they are trapped in reservations and have lost their touch with nature and ability to exist with dignity. They were chased off their lands and eventually forced to live lives in which they ate foods that were harmful to them. Alcoholism is a result of the oppression brought upon them and adds to the symptoms of diabetes. The truth is they lost their calling, their right livelihoods, and their destiny.

All individuals on this planet suffer because of the wrong choices of others who should be aids along their destiny paths. Instead, many millions of individuals are just looking out for themselves, not being concerned about being their brothers' and sisters' keepers, not even realizing that this is indeed a true principle of God. The false teaching that we are all gods adds to the problem of ill health. It is the height of narcissism. We are separated by religions, politics, and often the need for sheer survival.

The rich families of the world control the masses, and now in America, even to attain middle class, both spouses have to work without really understanding that God has a destiny for them, which is not just making money. Materialism traps us in a non-actualized vortex. We get caught in negative powers that speed us in so many wrong directions until we are sick, crippled, or dead.

On higher worlds of time and space cosmic families exist with the understanding of respecting elders who are our guides.

There is an authority structure, a legitimate hierarchy that exists for the common good of all. This is how a divine administration functions on higher worlds and is beginning to function with approximately one hundred individuals from various countries in Arizona in a prototype community called Global Community Communications Alliance, also called the First Planetary Sacred Home and Divine Administration.

I have seen individuals take a truly holistic approach to living—eating properly, taking vitamins, exercising, getting the proper rest they need, and even seeking a spiritual path—and still they end up dying of diabetes or different forms of cancer. Why is this? After acquiring the cancer, they went to alternative healers, some even to the best of medical doctors, but nothing could stop the deterioration of their bodies.

They, like billions of others, are the victims of poor choices by significant souls who should be a part of their lives but who have chosen wrongly and helped to cause the non-actualization of millions of their brothers and sisters. This is what rebellion against God and divine laws does. It may be at various levels of evil (which is error), sin (in which you have more knowing of your wrong-doing), or iniquity (in which you know you are doing wrong and you just do not care).

The most successful forms of healing are what are called morontia counseling and tron therapy. Both of these forms are given to a mandated personality from Celestial Overcontrol, to be taught to Destiny Reservists who have a true calling from God to become instruments of healing. Divine Administration has been applying the principles of both forms of healing for many years and has seen wonderful results.

Morontia counseling has to do with counseling the soul and the soul's astral deficiencies over many lifetimes of rebellion to God. Basically it is the rehabilitation of the soul; it is not traditional psychiatric counseling. Since we are what we think, an individual must begin to purify the mind circuitry by overcoming negative thought patterns and non-virtue behaviors. I, being an audio fusion material complement, was first trained to be a morontia counselor by a spirit personality named Paladin who is a finaliter (see *The URANTIA Book*, p. 345). I, in turn, have trained others, some who already had doctorates and experience in clinical psychology and other counseling modalities before becoming morontia counselors.

Tron therapy then can be applied to aid in the body's physical healing. Tron therapy will not work unless a person completely relinquishes his or her will to the will of God and is willing to deal with all negative patterns in his or her thought-life and personal relationships with other human beings. Tron therapy at this time can only be applied by the Mandate of the Bright and Morning Star, held by me and my spiritual complement Niánn Emerson Chase. When an individual is a candidate for tron therapy, celestial beings work with the human healers to force out of the body all viruses, bacteria, and dio matter that may be blocking the flow of blood or Ch'i energy.

Even these two marvelous and new forms of healing will not work completely if significant others (who are supposed to be helping an individual in his or her destiny purpose) have failed to meet their own destiny by wrong decisions and have not been willing to deal with their own sin within—basically being in the permissive will of God (instead of His perfect will) at various levels.

So, once you begin to understand that your health and the health of your neighbors can be helped by each right decision you make in your relationship to a personal God, you then can really become a healer. As you begin to heal yourself, you will begin to heal others. I am sure you have heard that line before, but I hope that after reading this, this truth is something you live moment to moment, not just something you have read or heard that went in one ear and out the other.

In God's kingdom there is no competition; there is only compliance with His will. His kingdom is just for all, and we all have a certain niche—a piece of the giant cosmic puzzle that only we can fit into. I could not fit into your space in the puzzle, and you could not fit into mine. Some may be similar, but no two are exact. We are all created uniquely, with our very unique destiny encompassing many experiences and changes as we evolve.

Eternity (which we are in right now) is ever-changing, and if you are not changing, you will be ill. I have seen many individuals experience extended lives (when doctors said they would be dead in six months) and live many years after, because they truly began to change. Perhaps if all the peoples of the planet would begin to change by seeking God's perfect will and serving one another, disease and death would be a thing of the past—just like it is on higher worlds of time and space.

Some Thoughts on Healing

by Niánn Emerson Chase

The Difference Between *Curing* and *Healing*

We are all aware that this planet is in dire need of healing. In order for the planet to heal, the individuals, the human beings who have caused its devastation, need to heal.

In her book, *Ordinary Times, Cycles in Marriage, Faith and Renewal*, Nancy Meyers shares one of the most significant epiphanies of her life.

> A couple of years ago, I had an experience that struck me, in spite of its familiar setting, and maybe even in some people's lives, its predictability, as odd. I was at the Newman Center Mass I often attend on Saturday afternoons. Still walking in those days, I had just received communion and returned to my pew, where I knelt, and after one coherent little prayer, began the interior jumble that forms my post-communion meditation. This was even more of a mess than usual because I felt panic-stricken. My multiple sclerosis was getting worse, almost by the day, and my resolve to cope bravely in a manner befitting my stern Yankee heritage was weakening even faster than my muscles were. I just wanted to get rid of the damned disease. God, God, God, I prayed. Please cure me, heal me. And then for the first and only time in my life, I got a response. I had never heard voices, and I didn't hear one now. Three monosyllables simply materialized in my consciousness: "But I am."

Nancy Meyers goes on to describe her own inner process of realizing how God could be healing her while her physical symptoms of multiple sclerosis continue to get worse. She realized that in her mind, the actual intent in her prayer was, "Cure me of this physical ailment, of this disease." That did not happen, but she discovered that she indeed was being healed, and that the *healing* process is different from the *curing* process. Now she is in a wheelchair and continues to believe that she's in the process of being healed.

People today really are not that different than the way they were in Jesus' time. Jesus dealt with thousands and thousands of people who would come to Him clamoring for a quick cure of their physical ailments. They wanted their physical lot in life improved, and they also wanted a meal thrown in with it. In actuality, *The URANTIA Book* tells us that Jesus cured only a few who came to Him, and out of that few hundred who were cured of a physical ailment, only a small portion were actually healed.

Today, most Americans and Europeans go to a doctor, or someone in the medical profession, to be cured of a physical illness. Sometimes they are cured, at least temporarily, when the treatment gets rid of the physical symptoms that they are having. Often the physical problem comes up again later on, or some other physical symptom emerges. They can go into remission at some level. Sometimes the patient ends up even worse off physically than before going through the treatment. What exactly is *healing* and how is it different from *curing*?

On pages 1836 and 1837 in *The URANTIA Book*, we are told about an elderly woman who wore a downcast expression, was much bent in form, and had come to hear Jesus teach. For eighteen years this woman had been fear-ridden, and all joy had passed out of her life. Life had just gotten to her, and she was literally beaten up by it. Jesus looked at her with compassion as He approached her. He touched her hunched shoulder and said, "Woman, if you would only believe, you could be wholly loosed from your spirit of infirmity." This woman "who had been bowed down and bound up by the depressions of fear, believed the words of the Master." She had faith, and "faith straightened her up immediately." When she saw that she had been made straight, "she lifted up her voice and glorified God." In that section of *The URANTIA Book* we are told that Jesus frequently delivered victims of fear, like this woman, from their "spirit of infirmity," from their "depression of mind," and from their "bondage of fear." The people thought all such afflictions were either physical disorders or possessions by evil spirits, when in reality the disease was only the state of their minds.

Healing has to do with a shift in the mind, in the thought processes of the individual. Healing has to do with some kind of personal encounter with God the Father. For those who lived during Jesus' time and were healed by responding from a soul level to Jesus, they encountered God through Jesus. For Nancy Meyers, the woman with multiple sclerosis, the encounter came with the spirit of the Father that was within her, what *The URANTIA Book* calls the Thought Adjuster.

In Ms. Meyers' continued healing, as well as in the healing of those who were actually in some manner touched by Jesus during the first century, the Spirit of Truth from the Creator Son and the Holy Spirit from the Universe Mother continued to coordinate with that fragment of the Universal Father to aid each individual in their healing. Healing is a continued process; it does not just come and then it is over and done with. Healing is a continued encounter with the Threefold Spirit of God within you.

That is not what *curing* is. Most doctors really are not in the business of healing; they are in the business of curing. They can go into surgery with a knife and cut out the tumor, but they have not dealt with the mind of the individual, the thought processes of the individual. For Nancy Meyers, her healing—which was a real and valid healing—did not include a cure of her multiple sclerosis. Yet she knows that God is still working with her, healing her. "Please God, God, God, heal me." "But I am."

Jesus' Encounter with Two Women

One of my favorite stories of Jesus' encounters with others is about when He and His seventeen-year-old student, Ganid, were walking one evening, and they met two prostitutes (*The URANTIA Book*, pp. 1472–73). The women approached Jesus, and young seventeen-year-old Ganid started sputtering self-righteousness. "How dare you women come up here! Don't you know who you are approaching?" He started berating these women and yelling at them in indignation on how they had insulted Jesus, and Jesus said, "Calm down, Ganid, this is not it." Jesus said to this boy,

> I perceive, Ganid, that neither of these women is willfully wicked. I can tell by their faces that they have experienced much sorrow; they have suffered much at the hands of an apparently cruel fate; they have not intentionally chosen this sort of life; they have, in discouragement bordering on despair, surrendered to the pressure of the hour and accepted this distasteful means of obtaining a livelihood as the best way

> out of a situation that to them appeared hopeless. Ganid, some people are really wicked at heart; they deliberately choose to do mean things; but, tell me, as you look into these now tear-stained faces, do you see anything bad or wicked?

Those two women, who had been beaten down by the world and who had made the best choice they thought they could make, given their circumstances, were simply trying to survive and make a living. In those days, if a woman did not have a husband or a family to provide for her, prostitution was probably the only way she could make a living.

Those two women encountered God when they encountered Jesus. For the first time in their lives, a man looked at them with respect and true love and compassion. He looked at them not as sex objects, not as subhumans, but as human beings with dignity and with a fragment of divinity within them. In that moment, born in their hearts and in their minds was hope. It was hope that they could truly walk into their destinies that God wanted for them. Then Jesus went a step beyond that. He dropped in on friends for dinner with the two women, and said to the wife of this respectable family, "I am sure that you can help these two women start a whole new life." He gave her the responsibility of helping these women begin anew, and they did start a whole new life.

One of the women died a couple of years after of an illness, but she died a happy woman who had some self-respect and dignity and knew that she indeed was a beloved daughter of God. The other one became a powerful leader in the movement to help bring healing and Jesus' teachings to others.

I recall a recent news report of two mothers who killed their children and then also killed themselves. A mother who does that to her young children has been driven to a point where in her mind she sees no way out. She sees the world as so unacceptable to live in that the only thing she can do is leave it. She's not about to leave her children there to suffer in that world, for who would take care of them? The world is too terrible to live in anymore. It is a tragic thing that the world had gotten to those two women and that was the only choice they *thought* they had. Somehow they were not able to hear the spirit of God within them, and they did not have any human being who was somehow able to reach them to bring them to that realization that there were other options and other choices. These were just two mothers; there are hundreds of thousands of mothers across the planet who need to hear another message and who need true healing.

An Inner Life Needed for Healing

We know that in order to heal, we do need to provide the inner environment for the ministry of the Threefold Spirit of God and the other living spiritual forces to work with us. Often that inner environment has to have the outer environment, and that is what Jesus provided for the two women that He met. He changed their environment. He first encountered them in their hearts and minds, and a shift happened, a ray of hope came, and then He got practical and provided the logistics for them to change their outer conditions. He did not just go on and say, "Well, I will see you. Good luck!" and leave. He enabled them; He empowered them to move into another life circumstance.

All of us have something in common with everyone else who lives in this country and in European countries and Canada. We are human products of Western civilization, of a corporate system, of an industrialized and high-tech society that has all of existence mechanized for humans and all living things on the planet. Most decisions in this dominant culture are based on the profit motive—very little soul, or heart, or spirit in any of it, and part of that environment is that constant rushing around.

Many believe they have to make all of these time limits. Many are always aware of the time on their watches. They find themselves rushing outwardly as they try to beat the traffic on the freeway, and they get impatient with the person in front of them who may not be driving as fast as they would like them to drive. There has been quite a bit of media publicity recently about the increasing problem of road rage. It is just an outward manifestation of the rage and the frustration that is happening to people on the inside.

People are also rushing around inside their heads. That is why a lot of people do not want to be still; they are uncomfortable sitting down, being still, and actually reflecting or meditating, because their minds are going a mile a minute. "I cannot meditate, my mind's going too crazy." *The URANTIA Book* tells us that Jesus never was in a hurry. That was because He was in the moment, and He was in God's will in the moment. You do not have to be rushing when you are in God's will in the moment, but our dominant culture does not provide a safe place for us to slow down and to develop an inner life. *The URANTIA Book* has a wonderful teaching about the inner life and the importance of developing the inner life, and how if a civilization does not encourage that and provide an impetus, a catalyst for the youth of the culture to develop that inner life, that civilization will crumble and fail. We see this happening in the civilization that we live in, which is simply a product of the Lucifer Rebellion.

One of my favorite authors, Madeline L'Engle, in one of her books, *The Crosswicks Journal, A Circle of Quiet*, says:

> A self is not something static, tied up in a pretty parcel and handed to the child finished and complete. A self is always becoming. Being does mean becoming, but we run so fast, that it is only when we seem to stop, as sitting on the rock at the brook, that we are aware of our own "isness" of being. But certainly this is not static, for this awareness of being is always a way of moving from the selfish self, the self-image, and towards the real. Who am I then? Who are you?"

In order for us to really discover who we really are within our God-given personality circuitry, we do have to have that inner life. We have to sit in that circle of quiet. If we do not sit still at some point and are running around busy all the time, we truly are in static spirituality. Even though it seems like there's a lot of activity going on, much of it is basically meaningless activity, getting us very little of eternal value, and certainly not bringing healing and inner peace to us.

A Personal Healing Experience

All of us in Global Community Communications Alliance are in an accelerated process of healing. That time of healing can be very painful. It has been a real struggle for me in the past years having to deal with the physical aspects. I am no longer able to daily ride my bike four miles or do long hikes up to fifteen miles, though I can walk up to about four miles. My physical vehicle (body) will not allow me to do as many activities as I have enjoyed in the past, but I realize that I am really healthier than I have ever been in my entire life. I am in a process of healing, and it has nothing to do, right now, with being cured of all these physical symptoms that I am struggling with.

I have always been a person who has moved fast through life, having six children, working (teaching up to one hundred and twenty-five students a day when I was in the public school system), and being a single parent. I moved quickly, managing a household and working in a profession that I loved. There is a place for moving fast, and we can get a lot of things done, but God had been trying to get my attention for a long time, because at times I told God how I thought things should be and what His will should be for me.

So, it was a wonderful thing that happened to me when I was bed-ridden for about three months. During that time my heart beat very slowly, and I could not even get up to walk to the bathroom. It seemed as if my heart was saying, "I am not going to beat any faster than this, and this is the way it is." There are medical explanations of why my heart slowed down, but more important to me are the spiritual reasons.

I am in my point-of-origin reconstruction process. There are a lot of things happening on many levels; this is a multi-dimensional process I am experiencing. It is happening first and foremost in my mind and in my spirit, in my heart and soul. The physical manifestations will come as I make those inner shifts that I need to make. I had to be slowed down so I could be very present to hear that small quiet voice of God, which really is not very small at all. It is quite loud if you are listening.

I needed to be forced to sit in that circle of quiet for a lot longer than five minutes, or twenty minutes, or a day. In that circle of quiet that I existed in for those months—lived in, grew in, unfolded in—I became more and more aware of that deep smoldering anger and resentment that was very much a part of me, though I thought I had gotten a handle on all of that. Being a person who has had a few past lives, I had chapters and chapters, layers and layers of experiences where, as a woman on Urantia, I had been beaten down by the situation on the planet. We women have a lot of reasons to be angry, but I am not going to get into all of that in this teaching.

I know for my healing during that time, my anger had to be dealt with because anger and resentment must be dispelled or transformed into something productive and helpful. Resentment is simply unexpressed anger, and if not appropriately and effectively expressed, anger can sit deep inside you and manifest in some form of physical dis-ease. There was a healing process that had to go on within me, as it does within most women on this planet.

Anger can be used for good when it moves us into a place of activity, good activity, activity for God. We need to become activists of the Divine New Order. We need to become those change agents, and you cannot just sit around talking about it. Remember when Jesus met with those two women? He was very active in helping them bring about a change in their lives. He did not just talk it; He walked it too, and that is what an activist does. In order to help bring about a healing for this world, the first thing a true activist has to do is bring about a healing within himself or herself and then help bring healing to other people, and it is an ongoing process.

What has helped tremendously in my own healing are the Father circuits (Father circuits with a capital F) of some of Celestial Overcontrol and my beloved spiritual complement, Gabriel of Urantia. I am not talking about "macho." I am not talking about that imbalance of the men on this planet; I am talking about the Universal Father circuits, which can be very strong and appropriately confrontational.

The people of Urantia need the Universal Father circuits as much as they need the Mother circuits—the Paradise Mother and Universe Mother circuits. We all need them both, and part of our healing is to come into a connection and balance with both. My intent is to continue to get this true healing, to be able to have the kind of mind that is in alignment with divine mind. Often I feel like I am too "human." I want to be the highest human, the highest perfection that God is asking me to be.

Jesus is the person who walked this planet as a beautiful and perfect example. He did have His human ups and downs, and *The URANTIA Book* talks about His struggles, though He did not struggle nearly like we do. He had His human mind, and He had His divine mind. We know that we have divine mind within us through the Fragment of the Father, through the Thought Adjuster. We have our human mind too, and my intent is to have my human mind fuse with my divine mind, to truly be cooperative every moment with that Thought Adjuster, so that all of my responses to individuals in my life are *responses* rather than *reactions*.

When we react, we get a little charge; someone gets on our nerves or if someone gets upset with us, we have some emotionalism about it. Responding in true love to someone is being able to get out of our own agenda and to have an emotional aloofness, not having that sense of possession or ownership with that person. That is why Jesus had such a positive impact with those people He came in contact with who were open and responsive to His gifts of ministry. He did not have an attachment to them; He just loved them, and He could discern immediately whether He needed to use His Father circuits with them or His Mother circuitry. He may have needed to treat them gently, as He did with the women I referred to. Or He may have spoken very strongly and confronted, as He often did with those particular Pharisees and Sadducees who were deceptive when He confronted them about their hypocrisy.

For each one of us, in our healing process that is ongoing (it is really our ascension process), it truly is a personal thing, and my process is not going to be yours; we are each different. You should never want to try to make your process like someone else's because then you are denying your individuality and who you are. In order for our planet to heal, a unity (not uniformity) needs to happen on a global level, but in order for us to begin to feel that union with others—that union of souls within our uniqueness and our diversity—we must realize that what we all have in common is the need to heal, and that it is going to be an ongoing process. We need to also realize that we all have the same First Source, and we all have the same destiny to be embraced by that First Source of All, the Universal Father.

I would like to close with a prayer that was written by an American Confederate soldier who was seriously disabled in the Civil War. This was taken from Michael Lerner's book, *Choices In Healing*. This soldier, like Nancy Meyers, realized that though he may have a physical infirmity, he was truly being healed by God.

I asked God for strength that I might achieve;
I was made weak that I might learn humbly to obey.
I asked for health that I might do great things;
I was given infirmity that I might do better things.
I asked for riches that I might be happy;
I was given poverty that I might be wise.
I asked for power that I might have the praise of men;
I was given weakness that I might feel the need for God.
I asked for all things that I might enjoy life;
I was given life that I might enjoy all things.
I got nothing that I asked for,
but everything I had hoped for.
Almost despite myself, my unspoken prayers were answered.
I am among all men most richly blessed. Amen

The Elemental Necessities for Healing

by Gabriel of Urantia and Niánn Emerson Chase

Introduction by Gabriel of Urantia

Self-pity is one of the biggest blockages to healing in many people. When their expectations of how they think things should go and what God should do for them do not pan out, they can get very caught up in feeling sorry for themselves, feeling victimized. What many individuals think God should do for Urantia is often different than what God thinks He should do for Urantia at this moment in time and space. Often individuals think, "I have done all of this for You, Father; why don't You do this?" This kind of thinking cripples people; it cripples their minds, and it cripples their spirits. "Why did you allow this, God? Why couldn't you have done this?" Some people ask these questions often to Christ Michael Jesus or to God, the Father of Paradise.

Think of Jesus and our own self-pity. When He was being tried and persecuted—not only physically but emotionally—spit upon and mocked, despised by man, Jesus could have said, "Father, look at all I have done for You; why, I have created a whole universe for You. I have created the possibility of ten million inhabited worlds in Nebadon." (Right now, there are more than three and a half million inhabited worlds in this local universe.) "Look at what I have done. And now, You will allow me to be mocked, despised, spit upon, and crucified by souls that I even created." That is what Jesus could have said. Now we know that He did not do that. He did not give Himself the luxury of complaining, which we do as humans.

One of the major problems that human beings have is giving themselves the luxury of wallowing in their own self-inflicted misery. They think it is OK to have self-pity. We think it is OK to be miserable at times. We give ourselves the luxury of being undisciplined and less than who we could be. We live often in our lower selves; we even live often in the animal states. We live often in falling from our higher psychic circle (which may be the fourth). In an instant we can do that and stay in that seventh circle for moments, for hours at a time, for days at a time, when we could be resonating on the fourth, or even the third circle of attainment, and of course even on the second or first [the highest level]. We give ourselves the luxury of falling back to the seventh [the lowest level], and in that seventh circle people can act from cosmic insanity. We are definitely not communicating with others in the highest way when we are on the seventh psychic circle. We are definitely not manifesting the will of God.

A lot of ascension has to do with self-control, which is one of the fruits of the spirit. Another word for self-control is temperance. We give ourselves the luxury of flipping out, and when we flip out we err greatly. The more we flip out, the more we get into sin rather than into error. "I know I am flipping out, but I do not care." That's sin. Then, it becomes iniquity when you know you are really hurting someone and you still continue to flip out. You are walking in constant iniquity because you do not have enough humility to say you are sorry.

Gee, it is hard to be human. It is hard to be godly. Being godly is the hardest thing we will ever try to be at any one moment in any time. The most godly of all stood before Pontius Pilate, stood before those particular Pharisees who hated Him, stood before many others, and endured their taunts and accusations. His dying words for these ones were, "Forgive them Father, for they know not what they do." To live up to that one—and then Jesus said that we can be *perfect*—wow! I have control over my next moment, just like you do; what are we going to do with it?

For some people, there may be a need for healing in the physical body and, for some of you, healing in the emotional (which I will call at this moment, the "mind-neural disruptions"). Or you may have need for healing in the spiritual, which includes your mind and your evolving soul. Some people are so blind and obstinate to their own dio thinking that healing will be impossible in this lifetime. It is very unfortunate for them that this is true, because they are needed to help serve the people of Urantia, and in their obstinacy, and in their blindness, they do not see. Jesus said that if you could really see, then you would say that you are blind, and hence then you would be able to see. But if you would say you are not blind, then you probably are.

Teaching by Niánn Emerson Chase

I want to mention just a couple of things from *The URANTIA Book* about healing. Just before our beloved and beautiful Son of God, Michael of Nebadon, bestowed on Urantia as Jesus—an evolutionary mortal experiencing the many ups and downs of life—Immanuel advised Him:

> As concerns the planet of your bestowal and the immediate generation of men [and women] living thereon at the time of your mortal sojourn, I counsel you to function *largely in the role of a teacher* [all emphasis mine]. Give attention, *first*, to the liberation and inspiration of [a person's] spiritual nature. *Next*, illuminate the darkened human intellect, heal the souls of [people], and emancipate their minds from age-old fears. *And then*, in accordance with your mortal wisdom, minister to the physical well-being and material comfort of your brothers [and sisters] in the flesh. (*The URANTIA Book*, p. 1328)

So, Immanuel emphasized the healing of the spirits and minds of people before the healing of their physical bodies. Jesus passed that counsel on to His apostles and disciples more than thirty years after Immanuel's instructions to Him.

In His ordination sermon that is found on pages 1570 and 1571 of *The URANTIA Book*, before giving the beautiful beatitudes, Jesus says, "I send you forth to *proclaim liberty to the spiritual captives*," first addressing the spiritual nature of people by giving them spiritual truths; then to "*proclaim joy to those in the bondage of fear*," next addressing the mental states of people, especially the state of fear. Jesus continued by stating that His apostles, after addressing the spiritual nature and mental states of people, were to "*heal the sick in accordance with the will of my Father in heaven*." He lastly addressed the physical ailments of people, and implied that physical cures may not necessarily be in accordance with the will of the Universal Father. He implied that true healing of the body begins in the psyche of people, in their minds, in their attitudes. Minister first to the spiritual and mental states, and then the physical ministration will follow.

Jesus proceeded to give the beatitudes which start out, "Happy are . . ." and are *faith attitudes* and *supreme reactions* to the love of the Father. In other words these beatitudes—beautiful attitudes—are patterns of the mind, and it is our thought patterns that bring us happiness or unhappiness. Many persons have discovered this today, approximately two thousand years later, and we know that our overall healing is mostly the result of a faith struggle between our spiritual minds (our higher minds and higher selves) and our material minds (our lower selves). Part of our spiritual mind, of course, is the Fragment of the Father within us who works to help spiritize our mind.

A Divine Counselor summarizes all of this on page 43 in *The URANTIA Book*. He says: "Health, sanity, and happiness are integrations of truth, beauty, and goodness as they are blended in human experience. Such levels of efficient living come about through the unification of energy systems [the physical], idea systems [the mental], and spirit systems [the spiritual]." True healing happens on three levels.

If just the physical problem is treated without dealing with the root of the problem—which often is a soul issue, a spiritual issue, or a mental issue of incorrect attitudes, lower emotions, and wrong ideas—then the physical situation may not really be healed. (Of course, there are some physical illnesses and problems that do just have a physical or biological cause.)

The URANTIA Book (Fifth Epochal Revelation) states that energy follows thought. Continuing Fifth Epochal Revelation indicates that after the physical "fixing" of a health problem, like cutting out a tumor, another or the same physical symptom can possibly return if internal attitudes have not made the shift into a healthier pattern. If you are not walking within God's pattern, something else will manifest physically, and that's what we are dealing with everyday within ourselves.

I would like to remind everyone of the title of this teaching, "The Elemental Necessities for Healing."

One of the responsibilities of a true spiritual leader is to point out what the dio problem is in a person's soul. When we do that in the religious order of Global Community Communications Alliance, we risk making an enemy, because *if* an individual is not really wanting to change, he or she either will stay here in the community and harbor anger and resentment, or he or she will leave. They may deny many concepts that they had experienced to be true, and even deny *The URANTIA Book*! They may deny everything good that happened to them while they were in Global Community Communications Alliance in order to believe in the reality they have chosen outside of Divine Administration.

Denying the divine truths and procedures that epochal revelation presents is what the Lucifer Rebellion is about. Lucifer provided another way than the road of ascension and the hierarchy of instruction that does exist throughout eternity. Lucifer provided another way outside of divine pattern.

Often physical illness is a manifestation in the body of that other way, Lucifer's way. People may have a physical or emotional ailment due to no fault of their own. For example, individuals can suffer illnesses caused by a virus or a bacteria, or people can suffer the physical consequences of an unfortunate accident—a car or plane accident, or a slip and fall. Accidents happen on Urantia. Some of those accidents may be caused as a result of error or fault in another person; for example, a drunk driver causing an accident and harming others. There are many other examples of how someone's choice out of divine pattern can cause physical harm to another.

Because of non-actualization of a person's destiny due to the wrong choices of others, disease often manifests in his or her emotional life and then in his or her physical body, because that person is not in his or her higher destiny. That's a hard one to understand, because that individual may not have done anything to prevent his or her actualization. The wrong choices of millions have placed that individual in a box. How can the person live in that box and be whole?

It is not easy on this planet for individuals to become actualized, but it is possible. It is possible for persons to become whole and feel actualized, not completely one hundred percent whole, but whole enough that he or she can be a servant, an aid to humankind rather than being part of the problem. If ascending sons and daughters can begin to see and identify their own dio-thade thought patterns and bring their thoughts more into the spiritual realm of divine pattern, then healing can occur more rapidly.

Confession before God and another person is important for inner healing. That's one reason why the Catholic Church implemented confessional before man (the priest) and God. When you go humbly to your brother or sister, your morontia counselor or elder and say, "I have this problem within me; help me. What can I do? I do see this problem in me," or "I want to see. Help me to see it," healing then can begin. Confession humbles the person and prepares him or her for the ministry of the participating angels and humans for *reflective particle transference*. You see, I cannot give you my particles unless you are willing to receive them. No angels can give you their particles unless you want them in humility and the spirit of confession. The reflective particle transference will come to the repentant ascending son or daughter, and it often can come with the laying on of hands.

Without the soul searching and open confession of your own error, sin, and iniquity, no amount of medical drugs prescribed by the greatest doctor on Urantia, no surgery done by the best surgeon, and no holistic alternative method will heal you completely; the problem will just come back and manifest in another way. Only complete soul surgery will work, complete soul surgery. Soul surgery includes morontia counseling.

Laying on of hands, which directs Deo-particle energy directly to the problem in the astral or physical body, can also contribute to complete healing. The combination of self-analysis, morontia counseling, and the laying on of the hands is called tron therapy. That is what tron therapy is. Morontia counseling and self-analysis involves you in seeing your rebellion, wanting to change, and dealing with your evil by admitting it, confessing it. Then the practitioners can work through you. Rapid healing can be advanced by the laying on of hands. Tron therapy is direct transference of the God particles in the angelic and human practitioners to the "patient" and must be done in the perfect will of God.

Therefore, true healing of the whole person encompasses many essential elements that involve the active participation of the one who needs the healing—analyzing yourself for harmful mindal and behavioral patterns and repenting of them, cooperating with the living spiritual forces available, and interacting with other humans within the standards of God, not of rebellion.

Our prayer is for healing to happen to all of you, the healing that we have discussed in this teaching. God bless you.

Living and Dying and the Accidents of Time on a Fallen World

by Gabriel of Urantia and Niánn Emerson Chase

Teaching by Niánn Emerson Chase

What is the difference between being cured and being healed? As I have stated before, most physicians attempt to cure. True ministers attempt to bring healing. Curing has to do with physical symptoms. Healing has to do with psychological and spiritual symptoms. Curing deals with the temporary—the temporal. Healing deals with the permanent—the eternal value of the personality and soul.

In a previous teaching, I pointed out that people today are not really that different than they were in Jesus' time. He dealt with thousands of people who came to Him, clamoring for a quick, spontaneous cure of their physical ailments, and some of those did receive that curing, but the majority of those who did receive the curing did not receive the healing. On pages 1632 and 1633 of *The URANTIA Book* we are told of a situation where 683 men, women, and children were spontaneously cured of their physical ailments, but it is also revealed that the majority of those cured did not permanently spiritually benefit from their cure. Only a small number were truly edified by this physical ministry, and the spiritual kingdom was not advanced in the hearts of individuals by this amazing cure.

Realistic Expectations Based on Mature Spiritual Understanding

How many of us, like so many in Jesus' time, expect a quick cure from doctors and other health professionals? How many of us expect an alternative healing modality to cure us of our physical symptoms of a disease? How many of us have been disappointed, and sometimes even embittered, when our expectations for a quick cure have not happened? What is our understanding of illness, of healing?

Throughout the centuries, wise and discerning people have observed that, when confronted with truth, it is in human nature to believe only what we want to believe and in some manner to deny that which we do not want to believe. Jesus' apostles did it constantly. They each had their idea of who and what God was and how He was going to help them out. When some truth that Jesus presented matched their ideas, then they grasped it. When the truth that Jesus presented did not, they either ignored it or rearranged its meaning to fit their mindset. And these apostles were continually being disappointed, shocked, and discouraged by Jesus' confrontations of truth.

The only time we humans consider truth a *confrontation* is when it challenges our established ideas of what reality is. If the truth matches our understanding, then it is an *affirmation. The URANTIA Book* states that if we are true truth-seekers we will embrace the truth no matter where it takes us. On this fallen world, revelation so often takes us into unknown territory—out of our comfort zones—breaking down the little boxes we put ourselves into. In other words, truth more often is a confrontation rather than an affirmation.

Many came to Global Community Communications Alliance with expectations of how it should be. Many grabbed on to the idea of living in a "protected area" and not dying but moving into morontia bodies through reconstruction. The passing of some of the beloved community members over the years impacted established ideas and expectations of what should happen at the First Planetary Sacred Home.

The vision of not dying a physical death and moving into a morontia body is indeed given to us in Continuing Fifth Epochal Revelation. It is a vision for individuals who are stabilized in their consciousness and mindset in the fourth dimension and above—the morontia levels of understanding and doing. It is the vision of a society in the first stage of light and life—of individuals whose ascension level is in the first stage of light and life.

We know that Jesus, when He walked this plane as a man, as an individual mortal, attained the reality of the first stage of light and life. Continuing Fifth Epochal Revelation also says that many will pass on by the death experience before light and life status. [See Paper 55, "The Spheres of Light and Life" in *The URANTIA Book*, on pages 621–636.] There are some who still die a physical death even in the first stage of light and life and even in stages beyond that. How many of us, like Jesus, have stabilized in the first stage of light and life?

Most humans who are advanced in their understanding of spiritual reality are still in the transitional stage of becoming a fourth-dimensional individual. How many of us still fluctuate in our thoughts and words and acts between our lower human natures and our higher ascending morontia natures? How many of us are indeed healing and are not yet being cured? In order for us to continue in our healing and to possibly eventually be cured of our physical ailments, we have to experience many deaths within ourselves—deaths of selfishness; deaths of pride; deaths of erroneous ideas, attitudes, and actions.

None of us understand why very wonderful and good people die before their time. We do not have all of the answers of why some people's lives are cut short and others live into old age. As I pointed out in a previous teaching on *healing* versus *curing*, I have experienced many loved ones die of diseases that they were not cured of, but they were indeed in the process of healing while their physical bodies were deteriorating. I know that my loved ones who have passed on continue to heal in their new lives on the mansion worlds.

I would like to close with a revelatory truth presented to us in Paper 154 of *The URANTIA Book*. On page 1718, we are told that Nathaniel and James Zebedee suffered for three days and nights with an acutely painful digestive disturbance. They were very sick, and I am sure that they probably thought that they were going to die. On the third night, Jesus sent Salome, who was James' mother, to her rest and, in His humanness, ministered to them. But He did not, in His divinity, cure them. Why? Here is what we are told on pages 1718–1719:

> Of course, Jesus could have instantly healed these two men, [those two apostles, Nathaniel and James] but that is not the method of either the Son or the Father in dealing with these commonplace difficulties and afflictions of the children of men on the evolutionary worlds of time and space. Never once, throughout all of his eventful life in the flesh, did Jesus engage in any sort of supernatural ministration to any member of his earth family or in behalf of any one of his immediate followers.
>
> Universe difficulties must be met and planetary obstacles must be encountered as a part of the experience training provided for the growth and development, the progressive perfection, of the evolving souls of mortal creatures. The spiritualization of the human soul requires intimate experience with the educational solving of a wide range of real universe problems. [And it begins here in our life on this world.] The animal nature and the lower forms of will creatures [mortals] do not progress favorably in environmental ease. Problematic situations, coupled with exertion stimuli, conspire to produce those activities of mind, soul, and spirit which contribute mightily to the achievement of worthy goals of mortal progression and to the attainment of higher levels of spirit destiny.

I suggest that you read these two paragraphs over and over—the last paragraph on 1718 and the first paragraph of 1719. Think about what is being said here. Reflect and pray upon these truths that may seem confronting to some of you, for they may challenge some of your own established ideas and beliefs. Accepting this truth into your hearts can help you adjust some of the incorrect ideas and beliefs that you have. Bringing these truths into my own being is helping me, and I am in the process of adjusting some of my expectations—some of my ideas—to fit the reality of what I am experiencing.

I do know and experience, regardless of outward circumstances, the presence of God. He (or She) is so alive, so real for me. No matter how frustrated or disappointed or sad or angry I get, I feel and experience God's over-riding love and goodness and power. It is His (or Her) presence and power that aids me in being victorious over my lower tendencies that would forget the divine and holy, the beauty and goodness, the light and life.

It is work, and it is conflict—this ascension, this healing. We cannot run out and buy this great crystal that is going to do it. We cannot have someone dust our little auras to do it. It does not happen that way, no matter how much we want it to be an easier gig.

I would like to remind everyone of the title of this teaching, "Living and Dying and the Accidents of Time on a Fallen World."

Perhaps for some, the concept "Divine Administration" implies that we humans might be above the sufferings and trials of those in the third dimension. Some may think that we do not have to suffer any tribulations since we here in Global Community Communications Alliance are divinely mandated to learn, live, and implement divine administration and fourth-dimensional reality.

Some people have thought, for whatever reasons, that death would not occur within the community of Divine Administration. Some even have come to Global Community Communications Alliance because they thought they would not have to die, that they would automatically move into their next, higher body, the morontia body, without going through the death process.

Some have even believed that some of the apostles of Jesus who have regathered in Divine Administration can bring instant healing of all diseases by a mere touch. As Niánn just pointed out, Jesus did not even heal His apostles when they were sick with something like a flu. *The URANTIA Book* says on page 1649:

> In speaking to those assembled, Jesus said: "Many of you are here, sick and afflicted, because of your many years of wrong living. Some suffer from the accidents of time, others, as a result of the mistakes of their forebears, while some of you struggle under the handicaps of the imperfect conditions of your temporal existence. But my Father works, and I would work, to improve your earthly state but more especially to insure your eternal estate. None of us can do much to change the difficulties of life unless we discover the Father in heaven so wills. After all, we are all beholden to do the will of the Eternal. If you could all be healed of your physical afflictions, you would indeed marvel, but it is even greater that you should be cleansed of all spiritual disease and find yourselves healed of all moral infirmities. You are all God's children; you are the sons of the heavenly Father. The bonds of time may seem to afflict you, but the God of eternity loves you. And when the time of judgment shall come, fear not, you shall all find, not only justice, but an abundance of mercy. Verily, verily, I say to you: He who hears the gospel of the kingdom and believes in this teaching of sonship with God, has eternal life; already are such believers passing from judgment and

> death to light and life. And the hour is coming in which even those who are in the tombs shall hear the voice of the resurrection.

Most starseed are victims of past tragedies and are trying to recover in their hearts and minds from those past traumas. All of us will still have many challenges and problems that we must face in our lives. We will continue to experience the disappointment and grief of losing family members and friends.

Misunderstandings Due to Taking Information Out of Context

The Cosmic Family, Volume I and other teachings from Continuing Fifth Epochal Revelation cannot be taken out of context. Continuing Fifth Epochal Revelation does not teach that individuals will automatically not suffer, or not get sick, or not die if they join Divine Administration. What Continuing Fifth Epochal Revelation does teach is that there is the possibility, and in the future it is the destiny, for persons to be totally healed of physical problems and not die a physical death, but just ascend into the morontia body. It is the probability when fourth-dimensional (and above) reality is completely manifested. That reality has not manifested yet, but we are in the process of creating and implementing the reality, stage by stage, precept upon precept, step by step, inch by inch.

You cannot take a sentence from here or there to prove an argument—not in the Old Testament, not in the New Testament, not in *The URANTIA Book*, and not in *The Cosmic Family, Volume I*—particularly not in *The Cosmic Family, Volume I* because it is just a continuation of a huge, huge epochal revelation. *The URANTIA Book* certainly does not teach that people do not have to die. It gives very clear evidence that in the first stage of light and life, there are still some people who cannot go into the morontia temple and transcend and get a new body without going through the death experience.

You must be able to see the whole revelation in context. And that is one of the problems with studying any kind of revelation or any kind of spiritual teaching—not just the Old Testament, or the

New Testament, or *The Cosmic Family* volumes, but any written scripture: the Torah, the Cabala, the Bhagavad-Gita, anything—taking a sentence out here or there to try to prove an argument from one sentence. You have to know the whole text, and in this case the whole text is *The URANTIA Book* and *The Cosmic Family, Volumes I, II, III*, and *IV*. You have to know it all.

We all need to see things a thousand different ways. We need to learn to walk in the mystery of our eternity, not knowing all of the answers. In fact, often the mystery is not knowing any answers. Even the celestial personalities do not know all of the answers; they too have to live with some questions.

Sri Aurobindo and Mother Aurobindo, from India, tried to bypass the death experience by living a righteous life as much as possible, to become as perfect as they could be. But they both died, and I believe they both died in their nineties, and so they both did live a nice long life. Celestial Overcontrol said that there were not enough higher ascending sons and daughters joined with them to enable them to transcend the death experience, and there was no morontia temple that they could walk into in their nineties. Even if it had been time for them to have a new body, the temple is not here yet. Or if they had fused with the Thought Adjusters, perhaps, like Enoch, they would not be here. Poof! They would be gone. So even if they could have done it, they would not have stayed here.

We cannot live in the doctrines of the many religions on this world. We have to live in the totality of the context of the whole revelation. Even when the morontia temple is brought to a world in the first stage of light and life, all mortals are not ready to go into it for their ascension to receive their first morontian body, without experiencing the death process.

Death and Suffering Have Many Variables

There is much personal responsibility involved in soul and body healing. Death is an awesome (and awful) subject. Losing loved ones to the other side can be one of the greatest pains in life for those of us who are left behind in this dimension. Individuals who lose loved ones often get mad at the doctor. "You should have done something." "You did not do enough." "You did it." They get mad at each other in the families. "You should have done this; you should have done that." "Why didn't you do this?" "If you would have done this, they would not have gone. They would not have died. They would not have gotten sick. They would have gotten better." Or they get mad at the one who died. "Why did you leave us?" "Why did you leave me?" "You should not have left me." They get mad. They even get mad at God. And they never talk to God again, some of them, because they think God did it. God took them.

You really do have to have a wonderful expanded perspective on death and dying on a fallen world, even on a higher world in the first stage of light and life. You have to understand why people still transcend by the death experience. There are so many variables, not one variable over here, or two, or three, or four, but maybe a thousand different variables. I do not know how many I have got in my consciousness, but I am looking at as many variables as I can look at. And I still do not have all of the answers. I am only a human mortal. Jesus said in *The URANTIA Book* on p. 1664:

> . . . The Father in heaven does not willingly afflict the children of men. Man suffers, first, from the accidents of time and the imperfections of the evil of an immature physical existence. Next, he suffers the inexorable consequences of sin—the transgression of the laws of light and life. And finally, man reaps the harvest of his own iniquitous persistence in rebellion against the righteous rule of heaven on earth. But man's miseries are not a *personal* visitation of divine judgment. Man can, and will, do much to lessen his temporal sufferings. But once and for all be delivered from the superstition that God afflicts man at the behest of the evil one. Study the Book of Job just to discover how many wrong ideas of God even good men may honestly entertain; and then note how even the painfully afflicted Job found the God of comfort and salvation in spite of such erroneous teachings. At last his faith pierced the clouds of suffering to discern the light of life pouring forth from the Father as healing mercy and everlasting righteousness.

Many years ago I had tumors in my throat, and the doctors told me that I would never sing again and that I would need speech therapy just to learn how to talk after they operated on me. I suffered from this for several months, not being able to speak in a normal voice, but in croaking, almost-unintelligible sounds. My words were not clear, and it was difficult for others to understand what I was saying. I could not figure out why God allowed this to happen. Why didn't He just take care of it, make the tumors go away so that I did not have to deal with this one?

I thought and thought about this, praying over and over. Finally, I knew that God wanted me to go on serving Him with a damaged throat, with the facts that I would never sing again and would need speech therapy to just learn how to talk with half a throat. I finally accepted my dilemma, and even though it would be like that, I would serve God. I would leave the music—singing, all of that—for the next world. I came to that decision, not angrily, not because I had to, but because I wanted to. When I came to that decision, three days later, I was healed. Now I am not saying that always someone's disease will be cured when they accept it and agree to serve God. I am saying that they will be healed spiritually, and maybe, just maybe, like with me, their disease will be cured too. But that is not always the case.

I do not have all of the answers; no one does, and as I said before, not even the celestial beings have all the answers in this area, though they have a lot more than we humans have.

Why do individuals die so young? What is it that maybe they cannot face? It is between the person and God. What you cannot face is between you and God. Death is not being put in the ground, never to be heard of again. You are eternal souls, and whatever you need to deal with for your complete healing is just going to be done in the mansion worlds, the next planes of existence after this physical world.

Sometimes someone's death is a choice that he or she makes. Often the choice is not good or bad; it is just a choice that is made. Sometimes the choice is a lower one, for the highest destiny of the individual who chose to die would be to continue on this world with a higher mission in service to God. Dr. Scott Peck, in his book *In Search of Stones*, stated:

> The time of human death is usually not wholly an accident; there is a certain slightly discernable interaction between God and the individual human soul that helps determine it.

Higher Cultures That Contribute to Prevention of Diseases of Body and Mind

We here are very few as Destiny Reservists in Divine Administration, and in many ways we are still victims of the wrong choices of others as well as still suffering from our own bad choices. Therefore we cannot be fully actualized. We are deprived creatively to use our God-given talents for His Kingdom. In *The URANTIA Book* it says about Jesus on page 1671:

> He dared to teach that catastrophes of nature, accidents of time, and other calamitous happenings are not visitations of divine judgments or mysterious dispensations of Providence.

I think that we in Divine Administration still live a very high quality of life—higher than any other individuals on Urantia . We talk and walk in higher consciousness with each other. Our children do not have to be harmed in spirit and in mind by the messages of the third dimension.

All responsible adults should notice what music children listen to. All of us should watch the videos and DVDs the children see. We should be careful that nothing from the dominant culture that could be harmful is brought into our children's existence, because their hearts and minds can be diseased by the influences that are based on selfish and materialistic motives.

It may take years and years before you see the results of disease, or the symptoms might show up in just a few days. It shows up in a general boredom of life, an underlying anger and resentment, an empty, permeating sense of despair. A mindset and value system that is outside of the truth, beauty, and goodness of God can lead to very harmful addictive patterns, habits that are destructive to self and to others.

You parents need to build higher cultures in which your children can be protected from the diseases of the dominant culture that so many of us had to go through and recover from. Become more discerning with your children. Correct and guide them when needed. Don't try to be a brother and sister to your children; be a mother and father. We can protect them from the spiritual and mental diseases from which we have suffered in the past. We can protect them from that pain for a while, but as they become adults, they will then have to make choices of self-protection in God's pattern or pain and disease in Lucifer's manifesto. As much as possible, we in Divine Administration do leave the false systems and values that cause so much pain and suffering, so much disease, mental, spiritual, and physical.

Let us practice preventative measures so that many of us adults and especially our children can have long, rich lives. We can give our children and the children of the world hope for the future of fulfillment in their lives, of actualization in their lives. We can give them hope for higher and expanded truth. We can give them beauty and goodness by living it. It is OK to be kind. It is OK to be nice. It is OK to walk around like a nice little fairy in the woods. It is OK to be joyful. It is OK to be neat. It is OK to encourage our children to live by higher standards of conduct and morality than that of the dominant culture. If our children pick up those lower standards of behavior and attitudes, they are not going to walk their lives in beauty, goodness, and good health; instead they are going to walk their lives in distortion, unhappiness, and poor health.

While growing up I watched in my neighborhood the acting out of the idea that if you beat somebody up, you were cool. You were bigger and badder than someone else. So we had some neighborhood bullies strutting around who were considered "cool." We do not want to raise bullies in this community. We do not want any of the children to be afraid of any of the other children. We need to teach our bigger children not to be bullies, not to manhandle others. They do not become "men" because they are bigger and badder than other men. Walking in goodness is not walking in machismo.

Walking in goodness recognizes the God in all of us, the humility in all of us, the gifts in all of us, and the beauty in all of us. That's what we have to walk in—truth, beauty, and goodness. We need to teach our children that. We also need to teach our children respect for their elders, and we elders need to live in a way where the children see the God in us, see that we do "walk our talk." If we do not do this, they will become diseased in spirit, in mind, in heart, and even in body.

In closing, I challenge all of you to become bigger than your lower self and walk and live in your higher self in divine pattern and law. Renewal of life and healing can then happen.

Rendezvousing with the Rainbow: Building Bridges to Higher Healing

by Niánn Emerson Chase

Recently, while visiting some of my family, I walked Dean Star Dancer's land and was saddened by the deadness and emptiness that I felt. During my growing-up years, Dean had been a close friend of my family's. As a child I would often go to her place for hot chocolate, laughter, and a good story. When I was in high school I would weekly visit Dean after school before going home. By that time it was I who was telling the stories and making her laugh, for Dean had become deeply grieved in her remaining few years. We had many serious discussions about religion, relationships, and reality. Dean was first a mentor to me when I was a child, and I then became hers in my youth and in her declining days.

After retiring, Dean moved from the Los Angeles area to her place near an Indian reservation here in Arizona. She had dreams for that place and for her life. Retirement for Dean was a rebirth, a new way of being and existing. She left one identity in California to create another one in Arizona. Most of the family, especially her children, did not understand her choice. Most were embarrassed by her and possibly considered her move as a mental breakdown, and after her death, her children had no interest in the nonmaterial legacy that she had left. They were interested in the material inheritance of real estate and finances, but not those personal items that reflected the move into her new identity and life. What was that move that Dean made?

She wanted to become more than she was. She wanted to go to the depths of her heart. She wanted to expand her experiences beyond what she had had in mainstream society. She wanted to embrace the legacy of her Native American ancestors and get back to dirt and plants and animals and away from concrete and plastic and machines. She wanted to find herself, for over the years she had become lost amongst the mannequins and masquerades of the dominant culture.

Her land became the physical manifestation of her own unfoldment. As she struggled to realize the depths of her spirit, her land evolved—plant by plant, stone by stone, path by path—into a landscape of little vignettes for meditation and reflection. Dean called her place the "Rendezvous of the Rainbow." At the entry was a little sign that stated, "Leave your worries, fears, and burdens behind as you cross over the rainbow bridge. Step into peace, power, healing, and joy." Two or three steps later a little bridge painted with the seven colors of the rainbow graced the path. After crossing the rainbow bridge, the path split into three different directions, each one leading to a simple landscaped motif that promised to take you into an inner journey of questing and discovering, if you were an individual of imagination and adventure. Unfortunately, her family did not have the understanding of the power of place, or any desire for vision questing, so they ignored the many little compositions that she so lovingly created on her land.

After Dean Star Dancer's death, the Rendezvous of the Rainbow lost its grace as a result of negligence and disregard. No longer did people come there to look for courage, power, peace, and joy. People with shattered lives continued to come there, but they were not seeking healing and composure; these ones were looking for enhancing their confusion and brokenness with the distractions of drink, drugs, and drudgery. Thus, Dean's brave new world of rainbows, rebirth, and rehabilitation was destroyed by those who were the offspring of the industrialized and technologized world of inner drought, dearth, and death that she had moved away from. Her garden of living soil, colorful plants, many-textured rocks, and singing animals became a graveyard of concrete-like dirt, plant skeletons, rocks turned to asphalt, and no animals.

Many years ago, Dean gave herself the name "Star Dancer" when she decided to compose a new life with more depth and purpose. The name implies expansion into cosmic thinking and being. The name reflects a newfound freedom in the joy of interacting intimately and lovingly with the natural world. Star

Dancer was a new name for a new life of adventure and exploration of the vast cosmos of outer and inner space.

The rainbow is a symbol of hope and life everlasting for many cultures. For Judaism and Christianity, the rainbow is God's covenant never to forget humans. The rainbow consists of the seven foundational colors that blend and flow together, thus a sign for synthesis, synergy, and coordination.

Barbara Marx Hubbard, a futurist with a hopeful vision, says the rainbow is "a mark of love signifying that the elevated individual is always connected to God consciously and is therefore whole, incorruptible, immortal and perfect as God in Heaven in perfect." Ms. Hubbard goes on to say that the rainbow is "the mental counterpart of atomic energy. It is the light given off by minds whose thought is vibrating at the God-frequency, consciously accessing the universal information system, consciously connected with the mind of God."

The Bakongo tribe in Zaire honors a rainbow god who stills the thundering storms in the sky and the violence found in nature and humans on the earth. This rainbow god is considered to be the guardian of the earth and sea, including the village and its community, thus he is the protector of all life from destruction and chaos.

Scientists explain that the rainbow is formed when water droplets in the air cause the diffraction of sunlight. I see each human being having the potential of being a water droplet that can reflect the Sonlight of Christ, helping to bring the rejuvenating and healing colors of the Universal Father's love and truth to our world called Urantia.

I do not know to what depth Dean understood the symbolism of the names she had selected for herself and for her land, but they meant something to her personally, and they meant something to almost anyone who visited her, for they are symbols that belong to all of us.

Dean Star Dancer represents many things to me. She is all those who have attempted composing a decent life within the mainstream and eventually realized that they could not be sustained. She is all individuals who have become refugees from the dominant culture of Western civilization—some of those have been able to create an enriching and sustainable life outside of the status quo; some have become immersed in the margins of desperate existence. She is those Native Americans who were relocated by the Bureau of Indian Affairs to urban areas for assimilation only to discover that they had been thrown into a terrifying wasteland of bigotry, loneliness, and poverty, experiencing dislocation that ended up in debilitating alcoholism. She is women who—having lived lives of constant interruptions from the demands of family, friends, and work—chose, in their mid or older years, to redirect their existence in their status quo of discontinuity to a new life of continuity and coordination. She is the mothers and wives who are abandoned by their families when they no longer meet the wants, desires, and expectations of their children and husbands. And she is much more.

Though Dean finally succumbed to her sadness and committed suicide (she shot herself one golden, sunny, autumn afternoon), I think that she had composed a life of dignity and compassion. She was victorious in recognizing that she was caught in a system of spiritual and psychological emptiness, and she had the courage to move away from that wasteland of systematic deadening of sensitivity and humanness. She did compose a new life for herself, a life of higher aspirations and ideals, a life of quiet and composure, a life of celebration and ceremony, a life of ministry to those who were broken and searching for deeper purpose and meaning.

I think that Dean's tender heart grew weary of seeing the devastation that the dominant culture wrecked on nature, on people, and on her own children. In her last days on Urantia, I think that Dean, in her discouragement and sadness, forgot to follow the advice of her little sign at the entry of her place: "Leave your worries, fears, burdens behind as you cross over the rainbow bridge. Step into peace, power, healing, and joy." In her depression, Dean did not cross the rainbow bridge, thus losing faith in God's covenant with her. I think that Dean felt not only abandoned by her family but by God. Star Dancer quit dancing on Urantia, but in her passing from this world she crossed another type of rainbow bridge that leads to dancing among the stars of the mansion worlds.

In our struggles to maintain sanity and sustainability on this fallen and pained world, we must continue to rendezvous with the meaning of the rainbow—a bridge to the mind of God, His fragment within us that is continually there to redirect our thoughts of fear and anxiety, our feelings of discouragement and despair to the reality of courage, peace, love, joy, and hope.

A Divine Counselor tells us in Paper 1 of *The URANTIA Book* that:

> The God of universal love unfailingly manifests himself to every one of his creatures up to the fullness of that creature's capacity to spiritually grasp the qualities of divine truth, beauty, and goodness . . . The divine presence which any child of the universe enjoys at any given moment is limited only by the capacity of such a creature to receive and to discern the spirit actualities of the supermaterial world.

We humans have two drives within us, the material and the spiritual. Our destiny is to evolve from material persons to spirit persons, and we struggle with much conflict here on Urantia in our unfoldment. On page 1199 of *The URANTIA Book* is an explanation of why it is so difficult for individuals to receive at times the ministry of the living spiritual forces of God.

> . . . in the life you now live on Urantia every [person] must perforce serve two masters. He [or she] must become adept in the art of a continuous human temporal compromise while he [or she] yields spiritual allegiance to but one master; and this is why so many falter and fail, grow weary and succumb to the stress of the evolutionary struggle.

Like Dean Star Dancer, many of us humans fluctuate between hope and joy in a vision of a higher way of living and the disappointments and sadness in experiencing the many limitations of living a material life on Earth. We become disappointed with ourselves, with others, and even sometimes with God if we think that He is not meeting our expectations.

I read about a forty-two-year-old woman who just recently jumped off a bridge, choosing that bridge to cross into a better life rather than her inner rainbow bridge that would have helped her have a better life here on Earth. A friend of hers shared that she had just gotten tired of living on such a messed up world; she became discouraged with all of the evil and chaos she observed. I think that she probably was discouraged with her own limitations too.

We humans also fluctuate between faith and fear. I have a sixty-year-old family member who is suffering from dementia, which is something like Alzheimer's. I have observed over the years her continual choices to succumb to her fears and anxieties rather than step out in faith. She believed in God; she attended church regularly and even participated in individual and group counseling throughout the years, but she refused to relinquish her fears; she was very attached to them and thus no change in her mindset happened. A relative told me that even as a little girl this woman had been haunted by fears, and she was brought up in a fairly healthy home environment with both parents present. Her family has watched a bright and beautiful girl, who went on to get a Master's Degree and pursue a meaningful career, gradually deteriorate into an almost helpless woman by the time she was fifty. Fear fed her mind and eventually consumed all faith that she had in the goodness of God and in the goodness of herself. An archangel of Nebadon tells us on page 556 of *The URANTIA Book* that "Few persons live up to the faith which they really have. Unreasoned fear is a master intellectual fraud practiced upon the evolving mortal soul."

I have another friend who, in her aging process, has succumbed to her vanity and is now in a serious state of depression. She basically has given up and quit living. She just sits around and moans and groans about the loss of her looks and therefore of her life. She was always a physically beautiful person, with people commenting on her prettiness ever since she was a little girl. Throughout her life she was very popular with males and always had them clamoring for her attention. Things came easily for her because of her physical looks, and she built a life based on materialism and outer beauty. She never really developed a relationship with God or a rich inner life because she lived in a culture that reinforced her empty vanity and materialism. Now she is losing that prettiness and feels abandoned, lonely, and hopeless.

Unlike Dean Star Dancer, these two other women that I have known have not yet made a leap in faith and attempted to create a new life, a better and higher way of living. Though Dean ended her physical life on Urantia, she was always more alive than either my relative or friend. Dean had become an artist in juggling the material with the spiritual. Though she had to struggle to make a living and deal with her own psychological demons, she never denied her spiritual nature and continued to nurture her inner life, thus continuing to unfold in her destiny. Neither of the other two women has yet attempted dancing on the stars or rendezvousing with the rainbow. But it is never too late. It is never too late for any of us humans to begin to walk into the primal mandate and destiny for each one of us—to eventually become perfect as God is perfect, to eventually become spirit persons living perfectly in divine pattern.

Though we struggle as imperfect human beings with our selfishness, disappointments, discouragement, fears, self-pity, vanities, pride, and lack of faith, we all have the promise of perfection within us. We can rendezvous moment-to-moment with God by crossing the rainbow bridge within; our material minds can meet the divine mind if we just continue in faith. My relative and friend, in the depths of their dementia and depression, can still become star dancers. An archangel tells us on page 556 of *The URANTIA Book*, "Stars are best discerned from the lonely isolation of experiential depths, not from the illuminated and ecstatic mountain tops."

Our so-called breakdowns, our moments of facing our own hearts of darkness can be the rainbow bridges that enable us to relinquish all of those habits, patterns, thoughtforms, beliefs, and ideas that are blockages to our moving into a new life of hope, joy, peace, purpose, and vitality. Remember, "Leave your worries, fears, and burdens behind and cross the rainbow bridge of God's spirit within you and step into peace, power, healing, and joy."

True Healing and Spiritual Growth are the Ingredients of the Divine Romance Between the One Healed and God

by Gabriel of Urantia and Niánn Emerson Chase

Introduction by Gabriel of Urantia

First just a quick note on an article from *US News and World Report* called "No-Fault Holocaust." In it there is a drawing of a little guy that has a little ring around him that says "moral compass." Underneath the drawing it says, "Absolutaphobia: an unwillingness to say something is wrong." The whole article deals with basically a Continuing Fifth Epochal Revelation concept in simpler terminology, saying that our society needs values clarification, that there is an intellectual laziness in our popular therapeutic culture that has pushed non-judgmentalism to the point of ridiculousness. "While moral shrugging may be on the rise, old-fashioned and rigorous moral criticism should be alive and well on many issues."

The article speaks of how the young people, especially teenagers, are unsure about their reality in many ways because they are taught that basically everything is OK, that there is no absolute truth, that all truth is relative. We in Divine Administration understand that one of the dangers of the New Age teachings is the idea that everything is relative and that there are no absolutes.

On the contrary, there are absolutes, and we who come into higher spirituality have to understand relativity within absoluteness, not absoluteness within relativity. In some situations we cannot live by the letter of the law, but there is the law. If there were no law, there would be no universe to live in, because everything would be chaos. There is chaos within order, and even that chaos within God's universe is orderly chaos. That is the relativity, but there is absoluteness that controls the chaos. Let us remember that.

I would like to preface Niánn's teaching with this brief commentary: Basically, everyone on the planet in some way is ill, everyone. We all suffer in some way from some physical ailment caused by either a physical outside source that has attacked our body, or by our thoughts that have caused the disruption of the circuitry of the divine energies in our body, and that disruption leads to some kind of illness. At various levels, we are healthy or unhealthy in our body, mind, and soul.

Teaching by Niánn Emerson Chase

I would like you to close your eyes for a minute and focus on yourself. Concentrate on where you perceive that you are ill—on a physical level as well as on mental and emotional levels.

As Gabriel said, you cannot help but be ill in some manner if you live on our planet, Urantia, because we live on a planet that is steeped in rebellion, and one of the consequences of rebellion is illness, broken circuitry, and lack of wholeness.

We here in Global Community Communications Alliance/Divine Administration know we all need healing. All of us here at the First Planetary Sacred Home are actively involved in our own process and are very aware that as we grow in our understanding of God, as the divine romance between us and our First Lover of all, the Universal Father, is extended through our growing and expanding personal relationship with our Sovereign of Nebadon, Christ Michael, we simultaneously experience healing in certain areas on some levels and at the same time begin to recognize other illnesses as those dio patterns within us come to the light.

In the course on *The Cosmic Family*, *Volume I* (offered through the Global Community Communications Schools), a study is done on how Jesus dealt with healing various persons and the masses who came to Him for healing. They needed healing at different levels. I want you to carefully reflect again on these words of counsel (that I have shared in a previous teaching):

> . . . I counsel you to function largely in the role of a teacher. Give attention, *first*, [all emphasis is mine] to the liberation and inspiration of [a person's] spiritual nature. *Next*, illuminate the darkened human intellect, heal the souls of [people], and emancipate their minds from age-old fears. *And then*, in accordance with your mortal wisdom, minister to the physical well-being and material comfort of your brothers [and sisters] in the flesh. (*The URANTIA Book*, p. 1328)

These words of counsel were from Immanuel, Michael of Nebadon's elder brother. Immanuel was giving Michael those directions and words of counsel before Michael bestowed as Jesus on this planet. Those words are almost the same kind of counsel that Jesus constantly gave His apostles. Those are the same words of counsel that we hear constantly from the Threefold Spirit of God within us, as well as from our elders.

As I did in a previous teaching, I want to focus on those words that talk about healing and how to minister to people. We in Divine Administration are being called to be the apostles of the Divine New Order, change agents, ministers. What does that mean? Immanuel said to first give attention "to the liberation and inspiration of [a person's] spiritual nature." That is the first priority. "Next, illuminate the darkened human intellect, heal the souls of [people] and emancipate their minds from age-old fears." *Next* is to deal with the intellect and the mind, and *then*, after addressing the spiritual and mental aspects of a person, "in accordance with your mortal wisdom, minister to the physical well-being and material comfort of your brothers [and sisters] in the flesh." Many in the medical profession, as well as most other people, have it backwards, don't they? They want the physical and material needs addressed first.

It was the same way two thousand years ago when Jesus walked this planet. About thirty-one years after receiving those words of counsel from Immanuel, Jesus was presented with a situation that He addressed. So often in their travels, Jesus, the apostles, and His disciples would be accosted by large crowds of people who were very, very needy. Many were seeking healing for their bodies; some wanted comfort for their troubled minds, and some really did want salvation for their souls. Large numbers of individuals were there just for the show. They needed to have a little excitement because they were bored with life, and nothing much was happening for them. They wanted something exciting to happen, like a miracle, or some great sign of power coming from Jesus.

He did not perform too well for them in that area. These situations came up over and over again, and even His apostles at first were some of those people who said, "Hey, come on Jesus, be a warrior now. Let us go after those darn Romans. Let us get rid of them. Show the people how powerful You are. Become politically powerful, and then perform all those miracles, so that they know that You are a Divine Son. Come on, heal all these people; You can do that. Bring manna from heaven. Be a magician. Put on a good show."

Jesus was not willing to perform those circus acts. He was not putting on a carnival. He would communicate that to His apostles over and over again, and they would be so frustrated because He just seemed like an ordinary man this way. "How can we impress anyone, and how can we be important if we are just hanging out with an ordinary man? We think You really are the Divine Son, but hey, You have to prove it." Things really have not changed that much. Basically, the mentality and spiritual understanding of the masses really has not changed much at all.

We are told in a section entitled "At the Pool of Bethesda," on pages 1649 to 1650 of *The URANTIA Book,* that the apostles and Jesus had gone to Jerusalem, and the apostles had been shaken up because Jesus had not performed for them or the crowds the way they really wanted Him to. A part of them understood at some level what Jesus was saying; each apostle was at his particular ascension level and understanding. But they really did want a show of power, so Jesus basically said, "All right you guys, quiet down. You need to control yourselves. You need to just go with the flow and trust me and listen to what I am teaching you. Listen to what I am teaching the people instead of getting hung up on the big show. Just listen. Be calm and relaxed." Well, that was difficult for them, and the Midwayer Commission tells us in the second paragraph on page 1649: "The apostles were somewhat restless under the restrictions imposed by Jesus."

Now, there was a pool in Jerusalem at Bethesda that was considered a sacred place. It was believed that because the waters looked a little different than some of the other waters they were healing waters. Usually there were large crowds of physically ill people, people who were really struggling and were hanging out at the waters, wanting to get into them, wanting to be healed. One of the apostles, John, used that as an example, and brought Jesus there hoping for a miracle.

> The apostles were somewhat restless under the restrictions imposed by Jesus, and John, the youngest of the twelve, was especially restive under this restraint. He had brought Jesus to the pool thinking that the sight of the assembled sufferers would make such an appeal to the Master's compassion that he would be moved to perform a miracle of healing, and thereby would all Jerusalem be astounded and presently be won to believe in the gospel of the kingdom. Said John to Jesus: "Master, see all of these suffering ones; is there nothing we can do for them?" And Jesus replied: "John, why would you tempt me to turn aside from the way I have chosen? Why do you go on desiring to substitute the working of wonders and the healing of the sick for the proclamation of the gospel of eternal truth? My son, I may not do that which you desire, but gather together these sick and afflicted that I may speak words of good cheer and eternal comfort to them.
>
> In speaking to those assembled, Jesus said: "Many of you are here, sick and afflicted, because of your many years of wrong living. Some suffer from the accidents of time, others as a result of the mistakes of their forebears, while some of you struggle under the handicaps of the imperfect conditions of your temporal existence. But my Father works, and I would work, to improve your earthly state but more especially to insure your eternal estate. None of us can do much to change the difficulties of life unless we discover the Father in heaven so wills. After all, we are all beholden to do the will of the Eternal. If you could all be healed of your physical afflictions, you would indeed marvel, but it is even greater that you should be cleansed of all spiritual disease and find yourselves healed of all moral infirmities. You are all God's children; you are the sons of the heavenly Father. The bonds of time may seem to afflict you, but the God of eternity loves you. And when the time of judgment shall come, fear not, you shall all find, not only justice, but an abundance of mercy. Verily, verily, I say to you: He who hears the gospel of the kingdom and believes in this teaching of sonship [and daughtership] with God, has eternal life; already are such believers passing from judgment and death to light and life. And the hour is coming in which even those who are in the tombs shall hear the voice of the resurrection."

> And many of those who heard believed the gospel of the kingdom. Some of the afflicted were so inspired and spiritually revivified that they went about proclaiming that they had also been cured of their physical ailments.
>
> One man who had been many years downcast and grievously afflicted by the infirmities of his troubled mind, rejoiced at Jesus' words and, picking up his bed, went forth to his home, even though it was the Sabbath day. This afflicted man had waited all these years for *somebody* to help him; he was such a victim of the feeling of his own helplessness that he had never once entertained the idea of helping himself which proved to be the one thing he had to do in order to effect recovery—take up his bed and walk. (*The URANTIA Book*, pp. 1649–1650)

Just from this short teaching, Jesus is saying there are many reasons that you have physical ailments, many reasons, and of course they have to do with living on this planet in its fallen state. But for some people who think they have physical ailments, it is a matter of the mind; they are discouraged; they are depressed; they are fearful; and the minute they can clear out of that, those physical ailments just go, and quickly. For others, there are physical ailments because of what they have inherited in their lineage, and this is what Jesus said too. For others, it is because of choices they have made in their living, unhealthy choices.

There are many reasons for being ill. Continuing Fifth Epochal Revelation states that now, in this time of the adjudication, it is God's perfect will for each one of us to be healed. But we have to choose that healing within the laws of God. First we have to be healed spiritually. This is the adjudication, and so if we are starseed or Urantians—no matter who we are at this moment—we all have things within us that need to be dealt with.

It is the state of the soul. It is our relationship with God, and we need to deal with that. We need to deal with those past choices that took us away from God. We need to reconcile with our God, and for some of us, that goes back a long, long way. Starseed have many chapters in their personal history that they are composing. First-time Urantians, first-light souls, have just started writing the first chapter of their personal history, for this is their first life. Regardless of soul age, each one of us human beings, ascending sons and daughters of God, need to move into righteousness. Righteousness means "getting right with God."

We people on this world called Urantia have so many fears and so many wrong ideas about reality in our minds, and those incorrect notions are results of the Lucifer Rebellion that has been going on here for 200,000 years. That Rebellion is part of the dominant culture, and so we who seek true healing have to move into a higher place in our minds. That is what epochal revelation is about, helping bring us into a higher mind that is in correlation with divine mind. That is why we in Global Community Communications Alliance study *The URANTIA Book* and *The Cosmic Family* volumes in the classes of the Global Community Communications Schools—to help lift ourselves up intellectually, to begin to straighten out and educate ourselves, reeducate ourselves, reprogram ourselves in how we see reality, how we see God, how we see ourselves, how we see others.

As we do that, it will impact how we feel physically. We who have studied epochal revelation know so many more things now that have brought clarity to our minds. Our focus should be on inner healing, and first and foremost, on our relationship with the Universal Father of All. All of the rest can follow if we persevere in following the counsel of Celestial Overcontrol, which coordinates with the Threefold Spirit within us.

Unfortunately, many of our minds are so filled with our own agenda, our own ideas and beliefs. In order to really heal, we have to relinquish many of our own agendas, ideas, and beliefs. *The URANTIA Book* says that we all have at least one pet evil that we hang onto. Sometimes the evil is just ideas that we want to hang onto tenaciously. The longer we stay in our higher minds, in truths that sustain our faith and hope of things eternal, the more we begin to recognize those things that have been hidden from us that can keep us from our complete healing.

I recommend that you write about the areas within you that you realize need to be healed and possibly are already in the process of being healed. These areas would include the physical body, your emotional state, and your intellectual status. How do all of these areas relate to your level of spiritual ascension? Can you discern the reasons that those areas are not healed yet?

If you have recognized some of those areas that need healing but cannot discern the reasons why they have not been healed, that is OK, just be honest about it. "I recognize this, but I am not quite sure why it is not healed yet." If you have those thoughts in your mind, with intentions to move forward in your own processes, and take them to God on a daily basis, change will begin to happen, especially if you also bring into your consciousness the truths presented in epochal revelation.

Teaching by Gabriel of Urantia

Music Lessons

I would like to remind everyone of the title of this teaching, "True Healing and Spiritual Growth are the Ingredients of the Divine Romance Between the One Healed and God."

In order for you to become the perfect pitch, you have to get into the perfect will of God, and that varies with each and every soul on the planet until you fuse with your Thought Adjuster.

We have learned that when the universes of time and space were created, they were sung into existence by the Universe Father and Universe Mother Spirit of each local universe, as they came together in complementary marriage and then created their universe and physical and non-physical beings. Basically, all matter was sung into existence. That is so beautiful, so profound. For some, it may be hard to believe; for others, it is the only thing to believe. In this great divine romance, there is the ascending realization that we all at some level are part of that divine orchestra.

The following statements are concepts that can be reflected upon for some time, for they each have much meaning. The union of two creates a harmonic sound. The growth of the two creates divine melody. Each note is a thought of purity. Each rest is a wise decision. The tempo must be decided by God the Father, the off beats and variation of the theme, by God the Mother. At any one moment within sixty seconds the soul can sing many different notes—majors, minors, diminished, augmented. There are consonant sounds. Within sixty seconds the soul, depending upon who the soul is, has a lot of different kinds of Deo or dio sounds coming from him or her that can either help that soul to draw close to a wonderful and beautiful angelic order of being or, on the contrary, to a fallen order of being.

The body is a crazed conductor, and on this fallen planet, Urantia, the body, as a crazed conductor, seldom hears the original divine song that was written very specifically and very purposefully for your individual soul. What the body does hear is inharmonious frequencies, discordant sounds, broken circuitries, and noise. Many people think that noise at some level is music, but it is not; it is noise. Certain forms of sound today that some people consider music and art are actually noise. It is very pleasing to the ears of those discordant, inharmonious, and rebellious souls, but to those of higher spiritual reality, those kinds of sounds can really make you go crazy.

Does it seem that your soul seems all too often to be going down the scale instead of up it? Now it is not that always down the scale is bad if you are playing a guitar, but when you are supposed to go up instead of down, it is bad. Knowing when to go up and when to go down—even just half notes or quarter notes—is very important. If God wants you to go one eighth-note down and you are going three-quarters up, you are out of divine pattern. If He wants you to go all the way up the scale and you are going all the way down the scale, you are not playing His music any more. As a matter of fact, you get so far lost that you do not even know what you are doing any more. There is the combination of playing artistically within the divine will, knowing what you are doing, and then there is just doing it for the sake of doing it, not knowing what you are doing, that has no rhyme or reason.

Pride causes disharmony and distortion. Pride. It blocks divine inspiration and takes the cosmic fun out of the dance of eternity. I have been a composer and a musician all of my life and in many past lives. In this life of coming across many musicians and people in the music industry at all levels, I could not figure out why a lot of musicians get together and rehearse and play music when they are so darn miserable.

Music is supposed to be fun. You are supposed to enjoy it. Even up and above that, it is the greatest high in the world. Up and above that, it is a universe high. Up and above that, it is a superuniverse high. And up and above that, it is a grand universe high. And up and above that, it is a master universe high. And up and above that, it is a Paradise-origin high. When it becomes less than that, then you are doing it for the wrong reasons. You are doing it for the money, for the prestige, because someone says you should be doing it, or for whatever other reason you are doing it. You forgot the reason why you did it when you were six years old. Now you are twenty-six, thirty-six, or forty-six, and you forgot what it was like when you were six.

The Musician is the Instrument

All too often musicians think they need only to master the instrument, and they can become the master, not realizing that they are the instrument. You are the instrument, not any physical instrument beside you. Thus Francis of Assisi said, “Lord, make me an instrument of Thy peace.” He went on to say, “Where there is doubt, let me have faith. Where there is envy, let me have concern. Where there is jealousy, let me have love.” It is a beautiful prayer, with much more to it.

I shared this experience with you previously, but I want to go into more detail here. In 1982 I had a tragic time in my life. I developed two tumors, one on each side of my larynx in the upper throat. A surgeon told me that I would never sing again and that I would need speech therapy just to learn how to talk again after they operated on me in six months. They could not even operate on me until six months went by because of the danger of certain things happening.

My hope was, of course, that it would go away, but the doctor assured me that in the hundreds of cases that he had worked with, there had not been one case where the tumors went away. That was really great news for me, being a singer. It was like him saying,

"You are going to die tomorrow," because I had written all these beautiful spiritual songs, and I wanted to give them to the world. I was devastated; I mean absolutely devastated.

When I left the hospital, I could hardly drive. As a matter of fact, I got a ticket from a police officer for going too slow that day. He asked me what was the matter, and I told him, but he still gave me the ticket. He probably did not believe me. But I made it home, and I went through several months of hardly being able to talk. Here I was a singer and a Christian minister serving God to the best of my ability, and I had just lost the person in the world I loved more than anything else (my second wife). I let my ministry and just about everything else fall apart.

I thought I had given God everything, and I said, "You know, Father, I am pissed. You know I have given You everything. I have served the alcoholics, and I have diapered them when they pooped their pants, worked with drug addicts all over the country, lived in conditions that hardly anyone would want to live in." I went through the list of all I did for God and what I did for humankind, the whole list of everything I had sacrificed. I was really telling Him, "Well look, what's going on here?" and basically His voice came to me very clear. At that point I did not know anything about my past lives or who I was. I was just trying to figure out who I was then, and what was going on, and if God was really real at that point, because if He was, why did He allow this thing to happen to me, His loyal servant.

He said, "First of all, Jerri (my second wife) is not your God. I am. If you love your wife more than Me, then do not talk to Me and tell Me how much you love Me. The ministry is not your God, nor anybody on this planet. I am. Although you have given Me what you think to be everything, you have not given Me your voice." I thought about that because I had silently, between Him and me, said to Him so many times, "Boy, if I do not get healed, I do not know what I am going to do. I will probably want to kill myself. How am I going to live if I can never bring this music to the world, never sing, never make the beautiful music I want to make; how am I going to live?" And the thing that basically came back to me was, "You have to figure that one out."

So months went by. I was still sick, still trying to figure it out. Finally I got it. I said, "Jesus, if I never ever get my voice back, if I never ever again even talk right, it does not matter. I will serve You to the best of my ability in whatever kind of ministry You want me to do. I will continue to serve the homeless. I will continue to work in this ministry, or You tell me where to go. I will do whatever You want me to do." I meant it with all my heart. You see, He knows when we are lying. But when I came to that conclusion, even though all my life since I was a little boy I thought that the music was going to be part of my destiny, I relinquished it, totally and unreservedly.

It was maybe the next day (I do not know the exact time, it could have been the next three days) when I got a phone call from a friend who said there was a Catholic brother who had the gift of healing throats, and he was coming to Tucson to be in this Catholic Church, and I should go, and would I go with him? And I said, "Absolutely." Up until that time, I had gone to people whenever I thought maybe I could get healed. I went to Mexico. I even went to the "Strongest Christian Man in the World" as he was advertised, who came to Tucson, and who prayed for me, but I still was not healed. I went to the 700 Club—you know, the whole nine yards; I went through it all.

Then I went to see Brother Pankey. He was a brother, not a priest. He was a brother of an order from Philadelphia, a very beautiful, humble man. I was sitting in the back, and the very first healing he calls out from the word of knowledge, and says, "Someone in the church here has two tumors. I believe one is on the left side and one is on the right, and they have been there for months, and you cannot talk. Would you come forward?" I ran up there as fast as I could get up there. I knew it was for me, just like I knew other things when it was God. I had been to all kinds of services where they say, "Hunda la tundala, chundala, punumbala." And then they grab you. "Yah ta woota toota," and they push you down and you fall and get back up, and then they are shaking you. I had been to all those things, and I never fell. No matter how big they were, I was always fighting them. Then they would get mad and give up on me and say, "Next." "This one is not falling." I never fell.

All Brother Pankey did was speak softly, and the power of God just came upon me. I had felt that once before at a Kathryn Kuhlman service, and I knew what it was, and it was happening. I laid there for a half-hour. I was the first one to go up front and maybe one of the last ones to go back. I woke up, and as soon as I woke up and got up, Brother Pankey said to me, "You call the doctor and you get it confirmed right now, as soon as you can, that you are healed, so that no doubt comes in there. Do not let Satan bring doubt to your mind that you are not healed." I said, "I am healed. Praise God. I am healed. I am calling the surgeon right away."

So I did, the next day. I called this surgeon. I believe he was the head surgeon of the University of Arizona medical school. Anyway, he said, "Your operation is next week. You do not need to come and see me. You have had the tumors all this time. I know they are still there. We are going to operate on you next week. We are going to take them out. Although you will not have your voice, you will be alive." I said, "I want an appointment tomorrow or I am not coming in next week." He said, "All right, I will make an appointment for you."

So I went in. The doctor did not even come to see me; he sent his assistant in, an intern. I told the intern that I wanted him to check my throat and see if the tumors were still there. He went down my mouth and throat with one of those surgical tools and said, "Well, I do not know for sure, but it does not look like anything is there." He said, "I do not know for sure," but I wanted him to say, "They are gone!"

He then said, "I am going to bring in the doctor because I do not see the tumors. (He explained that he was not a full doctor yet.) So I said, "OK, bring him in, please." The surgeon came in, with all his assurance that he was correct and doubted my faith. He looked through the instrument down my throat and exclaimed, "They are gone!" When he said, "They are gone," it was as if a ton of bricks had just been lifted off me, and my spirits lifted. I was thanking and praising God. Because I was a Christian minister at the time, I said to the doctor, "Jesus Christ, your Messiah, fixed this, fixed my throat and healed me!" He said, "Well, probably God had something to do with this." That is what he said. And I said again, "It was Jesus!"

It took another month and a half for my voice to come back to normal, but I knew it was gradually coming back, because I started practicing my scales again and singing, and my voice was coming back. I can tell you that it was like a new life. I had this thing with the Lord at that point that I knew we were OK now. I would give Him everything. It was quite a lesson.

The tool that God may want you to play may not be the tool that you think He wants you to play right now. He may want you to play a different tool, you being the instrument, and anything you do is music to Him, like when I was doing what I was doing in ministry. Whatever I was doing, I was sounding beautiful to Him. I was not doing what I wanted to do, which was always to play music, but I was doing what He wanted me to do.

So once you realize that you are the instrument, you have to ask Michael (Christ) which one of the local universe bands you should join. It is a big universe. If you happen to be from Urantia, your choice is only Urantian bands, right? If you are from a more advanced planet in the system of Satania where there is higher technology and space travel from one planet to another, you can hop into your little space shuttle and fly to another world and check out the bands there. "Hey, this is great, man, what is this?" "Well, this is called Cosmic Nip-a-sip." "Oh wow, that's great." So, there are different opportunities, but here on this planet you are limited. Either way, there is a whole spectrum of choices that you have to make.

Harmonic Complements and Humility

Each of you, in your own way, need to join a group of harmonic complements. Whether you are an engineer, construction worker, mechanic, gardener, or whatever you are doing, you need a harmonic team. At some level, not only are you playing a tune, but so is your work crew, and God and the angelic beings are listening.

You have to ask how you can complement your already written compositions.

Some of us have hearing power to pick up really unique and individual things at very high levels. Inspiration could be talked about for many, many days; clairvoyance and all those things are very complicated concepts, but for now, we can just simplify it and say inspiration is when you receive something to draw or create or write or sing or say or dance and so on. Inspiration is given to you based upon your ascension level—the inspiration you get from celestial personalities and various circuitries.

Basically and ultimately, whatever you do, someone always has done it before, so you cannot get too prideful about anything. You cannot think of yourself as too unique. You cannot think of yourself as too magnificent, because someone has gone before you in a higher world of time and space. No matter if you are the only one on this planet doing it, someone on another planet did it long before you. So ultimately, you are tuning in, and you have just created something that someone else has created once before, and they are doing it now a lot better than you. Now if that does not humble you, what will?

Once you have come to the conclusion that you need to become part of the already written compositions, you have to discern what part you are going to play in that unique blend of sound performers that you are going to work with. Whatever group, whatever band that you are working with, you have to decide what note you are going to play. Who is the leader of that group? You have to understand why you may not be the leader and why someone else is. You have to understand your place. You have to know your strengths, but you also have to understand your limitations.

As I have told musicians in The Bright and Morning Star Band many times, one of the hardest problems I have had putting groups of musicians together in bands is that the drummer wanted to be the lead singer, the bass player wanted to be the drummer, the trumpet player wanted to be the bass player, and so on. One of the musicians who played all of the instruments really should have been the singer, but he wanted to play the instruments. You may not believe that, but it just goes on and on.

If you get a breath of fresh air somewhere along the line, you find some musicians who really know what they can do, what they cannot do, and what they should be doing. Some of them think they are composers. Some of them think they are lyricists. Some of them think they are singers, and at some level they have potential perhaps for all of those things.

Potential is beautiful. We develop potential at whatever level that we can develop it. If I see potential in you as a musician or anything else, I will tap into the little piece of potential that you have, to help you to actualize it as much as possible as fast as I can. That would be God's will for you. But to think that you are here, when you are really over there, that's a problem.

Perhaps, once you have gotten all that together, beginning to synthesize all those things in your mind, you are ready to really be healed. (Remember the subject of this teaching—"True Healing and Spiritual Growth are the Ingredients of the Divine Romance Between the One Healed and God.") Then you will be ready to play the true music. And what is the true music? Well, on page 557 *The URANTIA Book* has a definition of art: "The high mission of any art is, by its illusions, to foreshadow a higher universe reality, to crystallize the emotions of time into the thought of eternity."

That says a lot; you could write a whole book on that. That definition is a human illustration of morontia mota. What is *morontia mota*? Mota is the higher spiritual philosophy of reality on the morontia spheres. Morontia is the next level of reality above the physical plane. True mota is not happening yet on this planet, which is material rather than morontia, but God wants to get us into morontia mota to make us true artists in whatever we do. To me, the morontia mechanic is a wonderful artist; the carpenter is an artist. Art is very diversified in its form and structure.

So the best way that you can become the divine performer and get into the divine dance and play the divine music is to develop humility in service to humankind—service and faith. Humility, service, and faith are the keys. When you develop those three chords, you can play thousands upon thousands of songs with just three chords. You could write a symphony with three notes and variations of it.

To really embrace humility, practice it, just like you would practice your instrument. You have to practice humility; it is not a gift of God. Humility is an earned discipline. So if you pray, "Oh God, please give me humility," He will put you in all kinds of situations where you have to practice it and be it, and it has to be for real. To pretend to be humble, that's false humility. However, it is better to have false humility than no humility at all, because maybe someday—in ten, twenty, fifty, or a thousand years—it will become real. At some point it will have to become real.

True music to the divine ear is what humility, service to humankind, and faith produce. That is the true divine song, with those combinations of the personality of God in your character and your instrument, *you*. When you become the instrument with those three attributes of God, you are pleasant to be near, and you become the piper of God for others less musical. Up and above being that piper of God, the Cosmic Troubadour, you have earned the right to begin to hear the variations of the true perfect pitch.

You see, the true perfect pitch is only heard in Paradise. All the variations of perfect pitch are heard from Paradise out to the one billion worlds of Havona, through all the trillions of inhabited worlds in the superuniverses, down to the millions of worlds of a local universe, down to the lowest of lowest of worlds of the new evolutionary administrative systems like our system—Satania.

That perfect pitch becomes less perfect as it filters down to the material level, so what a high soul is hearing with perfect pitch, believe me, my friends, you are not hearing. You may think that you can get closer to it with a machine. "Let's get a little machine together, a little electronic machine, and get that perfect pitch." If you think that machine has perfect pitch on Urantia, you are crazy. "Oh, it is electronic." Oh that's great, what's powering it? What is powering that electronic machine is a little dinky battery that does not have direct current to begin with. Nah, that will not do it.

Many times, what is on key and in perfect pitch and harmony is an interpretation of the individual. In your individual lives, some of you are more perfect to others than you are to someone else, so musical notes of a similar kind are written on the same composition sheet, so to speak, and maybe your note does not fit with my composition right now, but maybe I can place you somewhere in the total symphony.

Some of you want to be placed ahead of your time into the main orchestration all too soon. That is like putting a soldier in a battlefield to find if there are enemies out there when he knows nothing at all about how to be a good point. It is like putting young men into battle before they are trained.

My father, who was a soldier in the Second World War, said before he hit the beach as a Marine, "I want to know everything there is to know about the enemy before I hit that beach." He was basically a foot soldier with a rifle. He wanted to know what kind of artillery they had, where they were placed, what kind of machine guns they were using, how many commanders were on the beach. He wanted to know all that stuff. He said, "The more I know, the more chance I have of staying alive."

How do I relate that to healing and music? Oh, it is all a divine symphony, every bit of it. In order for you to become the perfect pitch, you have to get into the perfect will of God, and that varies with each and every soul on the planet. Until you fuse with your Thought Adjuster it will vary, all the way up to the sixth or seventh mansion world of Satania.

So I challenge each and every one of you. Many of you are on the road to becoming a perfect pitch as part of the divine symphony. I challenge you again to become more perfect, and even more perfect. Practice humility, service to humankind, and most of all, have faith in the reality of a loving, orderly God, who is the first and foremost divine artist and musician.

The Quantum World and The Physics of Healing

by Gabriel of Urantia

Those of us who study the fact that human beings have various bodies all functioning with the physical body should know that any one of those bodies may need healing before the physical body can be healed. Often, band-aids are put on the disease where deep soul surgery or emotional surgery needs attention. The physical body or cellular body has to deal with impure air, impure water, impure food, and bacteria and viruses. All that breaks down the immune system. But very few individuals realize that many diseases of the body are actually caused by impure thinking, in both emotional (etheric) and soul (astral) bodies. A series of negative thought patterns is called dio thade thought. This dio thade thought can disrupt any of the body's systems over a period of time and cause any of a number of diseases.

One thing that distinguishes human beings from animals is that we have more complex emotions. These emotions, when handled properly and in balance, can bring forth beautiful music and art and wonderful novels. But when emotions are imbalanced, they can disrupt relationships and cause actual physical pain to the cellular body. Many people fail in all endeavors of life because they have not learned to control their emotions. In the quantum world there are particles that need to flow in proper orbits with the neural transmitters in the synapses of the brain hence emotional outbreaks, depression, and anxiety all disrupt that quantum flow. Grief of any kind can also disrupt that flow.

Most people today work in non-sacred environments where stress causes the breakdown of the quantum flow. Americans work in a hurry, eat in a hurry, and, strangely enough, even relax in a hurry! America's workplaces are not really work-conducive for the quantum flow of higher thought, where deadlines are necessary, where inappropriate meetings are conducted, and where even meeting rooms—with lack of proper air flow and appropriate colors—all can cause emotional trauma. The environment, therefore, should be likened to a sacred temple. Human beings are all connected in a synergistic quantum way, particle wise, by the transference of particles to each other. So in realizing this fact, it should be more important to be mindful of the company you keep and not be in close proximity to negative individuals. A daily cleansing of dio particles could easily be done by coming to the Creator and bringing healing light energy through your body starting from the head and out the feet.

A new modality of healing called tron therapy is a much more extensive quantum healing process that eliminates obstructive dio particles from the astral body. The astral body is the collective bodies of all the lives that a soul has lived. It may contain hundreds even thousands of years of negative dio thade thought patterns. Therefore tron therapy cannot even be applied to a patient until morontia counseling is part of the treatment. Basically, the patient—with whatever disease—needs to be willing to change those negative thought patterns. Until they are willing to really deal with the root causes of the disease, only band-aids can be put on the real problems. Whatever the physical body has manifested in outward wounds in the cellular, the problem in most situations has started in the quantum world of the astral body.

The quantum world cannot be touched by human hands; it can hardly be seen through a microscope. Therefore only a healing practitioner who is intuitive and sensitive to the condition of the soul can really help a client. Once morontia counseling is received and complied with by the patient, various forms of other holistic practices can be additives to the expediency of the healing of the other bodies. The overall goal would be to align all bodies with the causal body. The causal body is the higher blueprint given at the beginning of a soul's birth into its first mother. On a fallen world, such as this one, the causal body should act as a guide, a higher chart, a diagram for intuitive counselors and medical doctors because the present emotional, astral, and physical bodies are far from the original design of the Creator.

Some individuals believe that they can tap into the Akashic Records and obtain this design, but in this wrong thinking, fallen beings will give false information. The causal blueprint can only be obtained through a right relationship with the Creator.

Therefore, God's will becomes important in any quantum healing, and the practitioner chosen must have a relationship with the Creator that is evident. Without the equation of the understanding of a soul being in the higher will of God, quantum healing cannot begin because it begins first in the astral and etheric bodies, which are both fused with the ascending soul. No physical healing modality—such as acupuncture, or raw food, or Reiki, or any outward healing practice—will have any lasting effect until the soul is dealt with first at a quantum level, and the soul lives in the quantum reality.

There is a saying that "it takes a whole village to raise a child," and this is true. It is also true that often it takes a whole team to totally heal a soul and a soul's body. This is because we are living in a world that is not conducive to holistic health. Ninety-nine percent of humanity never find their right destinies that the Creator has originally designed for them. Most of humanity, particularly in Third World countries, has to be concerned only with mere survival. In more affluent societies of Western civilization, many souls are led astray from those destinies by greed and selfishness. Greed and selfishness disrupt quantum flow of Deo particles and therefore Deo thade thought cannot occur. Higher thought is not self-serving; it is other-oriented. It is compassionate and altruistic. It seeks the good of others, not just in one's own nuclear family but the planetary family, and, as the consciousness expands, the cosmic family.

The most common disease on our planet today is the disease of non-actualization. The soul who is unfulfilled is a soul whose body systems, at the quantum level, begin to malfunction. Diabetes is just one of these diseases of non-actualization. Native Americans who were once hunters and gatherers suffer from diabetes because of the modern-day lifestyle that they have to live, and they accentuate this disease by alcoholism to drown their sorrows. Many other Americans also turn to alcohol and drugs to numb their senses because they have given up on their own dreams and visions. It is written, "Where there is no vision, the people perish."

Each person who refuses to be "thy brother's keeper" and who makes wrong decisions pertaining to the will of the Creator in service of others not only harms himself or herself but causes the unfulfillment and non-actualization of perhaps thousands of others, as we are all interrelated in each other's destinies. The Lakota term for this human interrelatedness is "mitakuye oyasin."

You have heard the concept "he or she has a good heart." What this means is that a person is a giving person, a generous person, and a person you can confide and trust in. The heart chakra (the heart circuit) controls the functions of all the other chakras, which also operate the various glands of the body at the quantum level. The quantum energy that moves all particles from subatomic to molecular to cellular is love.

Fourth-Dimensional Reconstruction Physiology as Opposed to Third-Dimensional Deterioration of the Body

by Gabriel of Urantia and Niánn Emerson Chase

Teaching By Niánn Emerson Chase

What is Illness and What is Healing?

As many are aware of, there are various reasons for illnesses and diseases. Many are familiar with rethinking the meaning of the word "disease" by separating it into "dis-ease." When someone is not at ease with himself or herself and with life, dis-ease can result.

Remember the story in *The URANTIA Book* on page 1649 about those ill people who were assembled at the Pool of Bethesda, hoping for healing from the waters. This group of people believed that the waters in that pool were healing, and so there was a group of them there waiting for the bubbles to come up so they could jump in and hopefully be immediately healed of their infirmities. One day Jesus was there and said to these people:

> Many of you are here, sick and afflicted, because of your many years of wrong living. Some suffer from the accidents of time, others as a result of the mistakes of their forebears, while some of you struggle under the handicaps of the imperfect conditions of your temporal existence.

As I have indicated before, often reasons for an illness are physical and social, and most of what some people would refer to as "miracle healings" by Jesus, the instantaneous healings that occurred, were healings of people that had these kinds of ailments. My guess is that the majority of those people who had those instantaneous healings were first-time Urantians, first-light souls (new souls who have not had past lives), and their illnesses were basically a result of living on this planet—through accident, through inheritance, through harmful physical ingredients being ingested, and through the wear and tear of living on a fallen world full of chaos and stressful situations.

We do know that there are many physical causes for illnesses on this world, but *The URANTIA Book* also points out that there are many afflictions that manifest physically that are the result of the thoughts and attitudes in a person. Jesus' words of truth in His revelation, if believed by an individual, could heal him or her. On page 1836 we are told that:

> Jesus frequently delivered such victims of fear from their spirit of infirmity, from their depression of mind, and from their bondage of fear. But the people thought that all such afflictions were either physical disorders or possession of evil spirits.

What thoughts and attitudes were in those individuals that manifested in a physical illness? One was named the *spirit of infirmity*. Think about that. What is the spirit of infirmity? It is thinking that you are sick or persecuted, that you are a victim of some past event or a victim of a present situation. It is hanging onto those ideas of victimhood. It is a constant thinking and speaking of how overworked you are; how sick you are; how misunderstood you are; how you suffer from what someone in the past did to you; how angry you are at men or at women because "they" (that other gender) have always neglected you or they have abused you in some manner. The spirit of infirmity is constantly thinking and speaking of how you were wrongly accused of something; how you were persecuted when you should not have been, and on, and on, and on. What a burden to carry!

Another attitude that Jesus mentioned was a *depression of mind*. Depression of mind is an attitude that the revelation of Jesus could heal if the individual believed in the truth and acted on it, but if a person did not grasp onto the reality of revelation, it would be much more difficult for an individual to be healed of this mental malady. Depression is something that all of us have experienced, whether it is momentarily, hourly, daily, days at a time, weeks at a time, or even months, or years at a time. Depression is a very painful mental state, but it is something that human beings on Urantia have had to deal with.

What is depression? It is a lack of hope. It is discouragement, and discouragement is a lack of courage. It comes as a result of being unhappy with the way things are. Depression can be a lack of vision for the future and a lack of knowledge and faith in God. It can be caused by being so absorbed in yourself that you are sitting in the dark cave wallowing in your own ego, pride, and self-pity. As long as you remain in the dark cave of yourself you cannot come out into the light of hope, having a sense of God's destiny for you and for the world.

Among many counselors as well as psychiatrists there is a very popular belief now that depression does not necessarily have a psychological cause, that it has a physiological cause, that it has to do with some kind of chemical imbalance. Hence, there are all kinds of antidepressants now that are being given to depressed people, little children as well as adults.

Continuing Fifth Epochal Revelation does indicate that there are many physiological imbalances and chemical imbalances that can happen, and often they happen as a result of thoughts. *The URANTIA Book* states that energy follows thought. So the antidepressant is not going to solve the problem; it may temporarily relieve some of the symptoms of feeling down and out, but it is not going to get to the root cause of the actual depression. Often medication perpetuates the problem rather than negates it. It is tragic that so many people who are in the field of healing have such a limited understanding of the human mind and the human spirit and soul.

Another attitude that can bring about illness that Jesus mentioned is the *bondage of fear*. Fear can keep us from jumping wholeheartedly into our healing. What is it that you fear? Do you fear ridicule or rejection? Do you have a fear of failure or of growing old, a fear of getting fat, or a fear of losing your physical beauty? Are you fearful of losing your identity? Is a fear of the unknown part of your psyche? On pages 1649–1650 of *The URANTIA Book*, we learn of one man who was delivered from his lower thinking at the Pool of Bethesda.

> One man who had been many years downcast and grievously afflicted by the infirmities of his troubled mind, rejoiced at Jesus' words and, picking up his bed, went forth to his home. . . . This afflicted man had waited all these years for *somebody* to help him; he was such a victim of the feeling of his own helplessness that he had never once

> entertained the idea of helping himself which proved to be the one thing he had to do in order to effect recovery—take up his bed and walk.

For years this man wallowed in his mental afflictions, his lower mind, because no one empowered him to do something about it until Jesus came along. What did this man do? First and foremost, he believed Jesus' message, and then he acted on it. On page 1905 of *The URANTIA Book*, Jesus told a group of people in His last temple discourse that "Many sick and afflicted have been made whole because they [simply] believed . . ."

What are we to believe in order to be healed of our physical and mental afflictions? We are to fill our minds with the revelation of *The URANTIA Book* and the Continuing Fifth Epochal Revelation, and we are to believe it in our hearts. We are to accept those teachings that are presented in this revelation as reality and not just some interesting concepts to intellectualize about.

When I first embraced *The URANTIA Book* and began to meet some people who had been reading it for years, I was shocked to realize that many of them—not all of them, but many of them—were not convinced that *The URANTIA Book* was a revelation and did not really believe that it was necessarily truth. It was intellectually stimulating for them, and they loved that stimulation. Of course there were those I met who beyond a doubt had embraced into their minds and hearts the revelation and that indeed it was reality.

It was another "coming of age" experience for me, realizing that people can get into a revelation and love the ideas in it, love the sound of the language and the intellectual stimulation of it, but not really accept it into their own personal being as actual truth that transforms them and their spirit. I was sincerely surprised to discover that anyone could come across *The URANTIA Book* and have that attitude, but yes, there are people who do.

Many of us here in the First Planetary Sacred Home of Global Community Communications Alliance suffer from various minor physical ailments. Many of us struggle with that because we have such high expectations of being healed and moving into a higher mind and a higher morontia body. We come into revelation programmed with ideas and attitudes from the third-dimension. We come into Divine Administration believing in a reality that our parents, our teachers, and mainstream society have given us. We come into Divine Administration with attitudes and ideas of instant gratification, self-assertion, selfishness, and the feelings of helplessness and insecurity. Some are afraid to believe that something wonderful could happen; it is too good to be true. We quickly embrace the messages from *The URANTIA Book* and Continuing Fifth Epochal Revelation of us healing and moving into fulfillment within God's will. What we do not expect is the time and the energy and the discipline that it takes to truly be healed and fulfilled.

Reconstruction Rather Than Illness

We all need to look at our physical discomforts now as manifestations of healing and reconstruction rather than a disease or an illness. We need to begin to rethink things. We need to think and speak something other than sickness and illness, because if we continue to speak and think sickness and illness rather than reconstruction, we will continue to manifest illness rather than reconstruction and a true healing.

Most third-dimensional doctors are going to tell us that we have a disease or problem that needs to be attacked by their physical methods, whether it is an anti-depressant, surgery, or whatever. And often those methods are appropriate and effective, but we need to look beyond just the physical ailments to the psychological and spiritual roots of any physical discomfort.

Jesus ministered to a young man who believed that he was possessed by a demon when in fact he was simply a victim of ordinary epilepsy. But this young man was convinced that he had a terrible demon in him. Can you imagine what it is like walking around thinking that you have some horrible demon in you? I would rather be an epileptic than demon-possessed. On page 1631 of *The URANTIA Book* we are told that this man had been taught that his affliction was due to possession by an evil spirit. He believed this teaching and behaved accordingly in all that he thought or said concerning his ailment.

When we do go to a third-dimensional physician or we carry in our minds an idea of what we have, and do not really believe what Continuing Fifth Epochal Revelation is telling us about reconstruction, then we (like the young man with epilepsy) continue to believe, speak, and act as if we have heart disease, or cancer, or diabetes, or PMS, or schizophrenia, or manic depression, or whatever.

Recently there was a write-up in *TIME* magazine about a study on PMS. The researchers took some young women who had never heard of PMS, nor had they suffered from any PMS symptoms. They split them into two groups. They educated one group of women about PMS—what it was and the symptoms. They never said a word to the other group of women. Can you guess the outcome? The women who had been educated about PMS began to suffer the symptoms of PMS while the women who were still unknowing about PMS rarely suffered the symptoms. Now that does not mean that PMS does not exist, and that chemical changes do not happen in a woman's body, because indeed they do, but it does show us the power of our minds and how our thoughts, attitudes, and beliefs can affect our physical bodies.

Continuing Fifth Epochal Revelation states that some of us can heal, that we can move out of diseases and be reconstructed if we are ovan souls, and renewed if we are first-light souls. We can all be healed regardless of our soul age. The definition of healing, according to *Merriam Webster's Collegiate Dictionary* is: "making sound or whole; restoring to health; mending; overcoming; patching up a breach or division; restoring to original purity or integrity."

The concept of "point-of-origin reconstruction" is introduced in *Volume II* of *The Cosmic Family*, and according to a glossary term of *Volume II*, point-of-origin reconstruction is defined as "the reconstruction of the complete memory and Deo-atomic structure of an ovan soul at the level attained before his or her incorporation of Luciferic thought into his or her circuitry."

In the definitions I just gave, can you see the similarity between healing and point-of-origin reconstruction? For first-time Urantians it is more of a healing that they experience, and then they move on into the morontia body. Paper 216 of *The Cosmic Family, Volume I* states:

> As the new morontia [light] body begins to create itself within the framework of the lower body, a great friction will occur, creating physical, psychological, emotional, and perhaps spiritual conflict.

We are also told in that paper:

> Starseed who find themselves at Planetary Sacred Headquarters and properly aligned with the Eldership, so that they can benefit in the spiritual ascension process, should find themselves at war with their lower natures and in discomforts of all sorts with their physical bodies.... Therefore, as you begin, within increased insight, to discover your potential and strive for that actualization, increased pain and suffering in your present body will be your reality as your old self dies and your new self becomes born.

My Own Reconstruction Process

Though I have shared previously part of my own process of reconstruction, I would like to do so again in more detail and a different context. Years ago I experienced some physical discomforts in my heart and lungs, and when those symptoms manifested, all kinds of other physiological things began to happen in my body. The stress in my heart and lungs affected (and still can) every other aspect of my physical system. If I had not had a faith in God the Universal Father and an understanding of and belief in the Continuing Fifth Epochal Revelation, my physiological processes would have been much more terrifying for me. I, as well as my family and some third-dimensional physicians, thought that I might be dying. Some thought that I had some kind of bizarre heart disease that most physicians could not understand. My heart did (and still does) strange things that are unpredictable.

There were times when I allowed myself momentarily to be fearful or wallow in self-pity. I think that all of us in our humanness sometimes succumb to doubts, dreads, and druthers. I think that in my reconstruction process I am truly dying in a way, and that is what Continuing Fifth Epochal Revelation indicates, that healing and reconstruction seem like a death process. There are certain physical aspects that seem to be deteriorating, and I believe that they are supposed to in order for the morontia aspect to be born, to evolve. My heart has changed its rhythm and rhyme because I have had a change of heart in my understanding of reality.

According to *The Cosmic Family* volumes, this experiment we are a part of is new, not only for us here on Urantia, but for most of the personalities in the grand universe. So, they are checking us out, and as far as I can understand from Continuing Fifth Epochal Revelation, this type of reconstruction process in material mortal bodies is the first time it is happening on this planet—this whole idea of moving into a morontia body without fusing first with your Thought Adjuster or going to the morontia temple and being reconstructed in that way, as *The URANTIA Book* describes.

This experiment is a new thing. Can you imagine the thoughts of the celestial beings that are observing and taking notes? We should always remember that we have these celestial beings that are right here with us; they are part of this experiment in some way. In my highest understanding I know this, regardless of the tremendous changes that I have gone through physically.

As a result of the changes that I went through, there are many things that I cannot do now that I used to love doing. I currently live in a body now that is no longer the body that I used to have. There were times that I grumbled and mumbled and sniveled and got frustrated. There were times I shook my fist at God, though those moments decreased as I adapted to my new set of circumstances. In my highest knowing, I now realize that as a result of the discomforts I experienced—and it was very uncomfortable (sometimes I felt like I was being pulled through a keyhole; sometimes it felt as if I was being turned inside out)—I am the healthiest I have ever been, even though I can no longer do physically a lot of what I used to do.

I used to do long hikes, fifteen mile hikes. I loved climbing mountains; I loved being physical. Growing up in Arizona, the heat used to rarely bother me, and now, I cannot tolerate the heat. (I think Celano, my planet of origin, was fairly cool, because I immediately suffer serious physical consequences if I let my body temperature get up to a certain point.) I used to feel like a real wimp, and at times I looked at myself as an invalid, but I outgrew all of that. Now I realize that in my reconstruction process I am becoming more powerful, but it is a different kind of power, a Deo power of increasing humility, compassion, and conviction. I have changed and continue to change.

So, today, instead of doing those long fifteen-mile hikes, I walk two to four miles, swim laps, do yoga and stretch exercises, and lightly work out on weights. I work full-time, actually more than full-time, and have a very active social life. I pace myself and make sure I get sufficient rest and healthy food.

I have in the past, during brief neurotic moments, made the error of thinking and speaking as if I had a disease or an illness. In my higher mind I realized that I was not ill, that I was (and still am) going through a reconstruction process, a healing. I think that it is so important that we all pull ourselves up out of fear and self-pity and wrong thinking into a higher realization that we are being renewed, if any of us want to be truly healed.

Perceptions of Healing and Reconstruction in Divine Administration

I do not have any "heart problems," and I do not have any "lung problems." I am just being reconstructed. Interestingly, my X-rays and other tests indicate that my lungs and heart are very healthy with no damage, etc. They look normal. And yet, I experience symptoms that seem abnormal to me. That's just how my reconstruction process is manifesting; other people's process will manifest in other ways, with other physical symptoms. There are so many levels on which this happens. On one level, you are manifesting your reconstruction in a physical way, probably as it runs in your family because you do inherit some of those physical things from your family. But remember, you inherit other things too, and for first-light Urantians you often have extraterrestrial genetics. Some of you are encoded, and of course for us starseed, we are learning to understand cosmic genetics. We starseed carry them lifetime after lifetime; we carry layers and layers and layers of what we have inherited.

Consider, when you feel like you might be dying or going blind or going deaf or whatever, that you are really dying to your old body, to your old mind with all of those fears, to a "spirit of infirmity" that you carried around; you are dying to all of that. You are developing a morontia ear; you are developing morontia eyes; you are developing new circuitry within you. We are also told in Continuing Fifth Epochal Revelation, in *The Cosmic Family, Volumes II* and *III*, that some of our organs within our bodies will actually just sort of go away, and some will be transformed and changed, so we have to understand that too. It is a very exciting thing that we are going through.

We are deteriorating to everything that is Luciferic, and everything that we accepted into our belief system and into our reality that was Luciferic. That is what is deteriorating and dying, but we are being renewed, reconstructed, reborn, rebuilt—however you want to say it. This "redoing" happens first and foremost in the mind and then in the body. Think of it this way too: we are in a living morontia temple, and we are not going to sleep and three days later wake up with this new morontia body.

What we are doing is a much slower process, but it is a much more exciting process. What an honor and privilege it is to be involved in it! We are transforming moment to moment—ultimaton by ultimaton, atom by atom, molecule by molecule, cell by cell. We are transforming organ by organ, and it is a very exciting thing. So, our renewal and healing does not have to be as physically uncomfortable as we make it; our minds can make it a lot easier or a lot more difficult. It is up to each of us.

I can honestly state that I think I am physically, psychologically, and spiritually healthier than I have ever been, and I look forward to continuing in this wonderful reconstruction and ascension.

In Closing

Michael, as the Son of Man (Jesus), became the true Physician, the true Soul Surgeon of Urantia. When Jesus left Urantia, He asked His apostles and disciples to follow His example and to do even greater things than He did. Before we can become those true physicians, we need to follow our Elder Brother Jesus' words of counsel: "Physician, heal thyself."

Teaching by Gabriel of Urantia

Fourth-Dimensional Versus Third-Dimensional Healing

I would like to remind everyone of the title of this teaching, "Fourth-Dimensional Reconstruction Physiology as Opposed to Third-Dimensional Deterioration of the Body." Fourth-dimensional reality is only being activated here at the First Planetary Sacred Home within Divine Administration. This is happening particularly for those individuals within the third psychic circle and above, which many have reached and stabilized on. How difficult it is to stabilize on the third psychic circle, and the stabilization for Urantians and the stabilization for starseed are two different things. It seems that starseed are held more accountable before God for what they know, and this all has to do with healing; that is the basis of fourth-dimensional reconstruction.

We are like holy pigeons in the laboratories of the higher celestial orders who are our celestial doctors. We are in an experiment on this planet, we starseed and Urantians here in the fourth dimension of Divine Administration, walking in an almost-near-morontia reality.

As Niánn was saying, we in Divine Administration who will be coming out of the third dimension will develop the symptoms of various diseases. These symptoms are results of patterns we developed in our lower reality, in our third-dimensional, lower-thinking processes. We are just bringing ourselves into the fourth dimension, and those patterns of our old, lower order are beginning to manifest symptoms a lot faster.

Some in Global Community Communications Alliance began to develop those physical symptoms before they joined the community. They knew that they had some problems, or they were diagnosed with a particular illness. Some of them had never gone to doctors for fear of what they would be told. Some might have foolishly thought that those symptoms would go away instantly or that maybe they could just go to the next healers' manual and search for the perfect New-Age remedy.

This is the generation of multi-vitamins and Spirulina. (It almost sounds like *Spiritualution*SM.) There is a parade of products that are supposed to bring instant health and healing—miracle pills to lose weight, "Vigor-ex," "MSN," "BCA stack," body-building products, hormone pills, "Polyenzyme A," "Slim-naturals," "Cleanse Smart" in five easy-to-swallow capsules, "Iprical Plus," "better than calcium alone," "Ipriflowing." The list just goes on and on.

"Until I found the cancer treatment of all cancer treatments I was neurotic." I guess so. The "Atkins Diet Shake." "That is what I like man, give me a shake, I will go on a diet any day." "Defy hair loss with new 'Shinmen'." Sounds like a Chinese drink to me. Anyway it goes on, and on, and on. You can just about find anything on the market that claims to take care of your ailments.

Then of course there are the healers themselves—and I have talked about this before. Beware of the person who calls himself or herself a "healer." Beware, because healing is not an easy thing. That is why I do not use *tron therapy*, even with Niánn. I used tron therapy on her eye; she was not healed overnight. I have the Mandate of the Bright and Morning Star, and I used tron therapy. I had all the Elders come over, and I was humbled because it did not work. It did not work as fast as I wanted it to work. She still does not have the sight in her one eye. I tried tron therapy on her lungs; it did not work. I tried tron therapy on her heart, and as far as I know, it did not work. So, there are reasons why it does not work. The reasons why it does not work for Niánn may be much different than the reasons why it does not work for someone else. If it does work, then there is a reason why it does work, but it is not all so easy to explain why it works for one and not for the other. Not one of us humans has all of the answers.

Some think that all they need to do is go to a holy man or woman, a healer, to be healed, and some of the Caligastia healers [people who take their power from ungodly sources] do "cure" you of the symptoms temporarily. However, the root of that problem will come back to you again, or a "sister/brother disease" that is close to its nature will emerge in some other place in your body. You cannot just remove the symptoms for six months, for a year, or two years, or five years, because the real problem is still there and will manifest in some manner.

Most doctors are aware that this happens quite often. Certain cancers go into remission for a while and then come back. With some people, a cancer might go into remission and never return, but some other kind of cancer surfaces.

Many think that the same spiritual concepts have various terms that are used by teachers of different religions. For example, "kundalini energy" could possibly be equated with the "antakarana," or the "Ch'i", or the circuitry of what Continuing Fifth Epochal Revelation refers to as a "central circuitry." Superficially all of these terms seem to be about the same thing; however, Continuing Fifth Epochal Revelation introduces the sub-circuitries—a subject that is so in depth that it takes decades to study the sub-circuitry of the various chakras in the body, what Continuing Fifth Epochal Revelation refers to as "circuits." So the central circuitry of a mortal is more than just the kundalini or Ch'i energy, and it requires an intricate and advanced technological cosmic insight that only can come through epochal revelation to realize this.

Healing Through Embracing and Living Epochal Revelation

At this time, it is only through epochal revelation that you can glean, learn, and understand new concepts that Celestial Overcontrol decides to give to humans on any one particular planet. The only way you are going to learn those concepts is to forget about Buddhism, forget about Hinduism, forget about Catholicism, forget about all the "isms." Take the truth that has been revealed in those "isms" and choose to continue to ascend with epochal revelation that is an expansion on those truths, or else you stay in those lower evolutionary mindsets.

In the *Kung Fu* television series that was popular many years ago, the wise elder mentor called his student "Grasshopper." That is what the student was in his understanding of reality, a grasshopper, until he grew in knowledge and wisdom. If you do not get out of your established evolutionary religious mindset, you will continue to be a grasshopper. It is hard to get out of those mindsets because those mindsets carry with them a certain kind of seeming spiritual holiness and a dio power with them. It is so easy to remain in the smaller mindset that has the millions of followers. You forget that Jesus only had twelve apostles, and He was the Creator Son of the universe. Many who said "Yes, we understand your epochal revelation," the very next day said, "Crucify Him," because being against Jesus was the easier route.

So coming into epochal revelation takes a lot of conviction and courage. That is why Cosmic and Urantian Reservists need to be of a special powerful Deo breed. Those who align with Divine Administration in the implementation of epochal revelation are in the "spiritual Olympics." They are the Marines, the Green Berets. Forgive me for using these military terms, but they are understood expressions on this planet.

The best of the light warriors, that is who God is calling here to Global Community Communications Alliance, to the Religious Order, to the Global Community Communications Schools—those who can not only come here but can stay. Many come and try to make it in Divine Administration, but they do not realize how hard it is to stay and be really healed. All of us humans have picked up those third-dimensional diseases in our bodies because of the thinking that we have been in for so many years, and we have a better chance of extending our lives through true healing in Divine Administration than we do outside of it.

One of my roles in aiding a person in his or her healing is to be a soul surgeon, to point out some of the root issues that cause psychological and physical problems as well as spiritual flatness and stagnation. Some people resent receiving information that addresses their deep issues; some people have a love/hate relationship with me because of this. I understand that. Many people had a love/hate relationship with Jesus Christ, and that is why they could say "I love you" to Him and the next day scream, "Crucify Him!"

Complexity of the Human Being

The soul is such a very complicated piece of morontia/spirit machinery. (In this context I am referring to the soul as the whole person.) I am always amazed when I learn something new about the soul. I have been around a long time, yet, I am humbled every time a new revelation comes to me about the soul, and I say, "Wow Father, I am so stupid. Why didn't I see that before? Why didn't You show me that before? Why is it that these insights only come at certain moments and certain points in my evolution? Maybe that should have come to me twenty years ago. Would I have been a better teacher for it?"

You are a piece of morontian-becoming-spiritual machinery who thinks, and feels, and has free-will choice. You are not meant to come into existence as a machine that dies out like a cheap watch. You are something that is built to last forever, to grow stronger. Your machine is not meant to become weaker due to rebellion; that is what rebellion does to you. What God designed, from the beginning, is that the mechanism, *you*—the soul, the spirit fusion, that which makes you who you are, the fusion of God and humanity and will—would last for eternity. The fusion of the Thought Adjuster and *you* is to continue to become healthier.

What Caligastia does and the Rebellion tells *you* is that you are sick. Many doctors in the third dimension make their millions telling you that you are sick. If you are sick, then those doctors can get a yacht. If you are sick, they can buy a Jaguar (or at least make payments on the one they already have). If you are sick, they can send their kids to Harvard instead of the community college down the street. So some doctors want you to remain sick in order to support their life style.

There are, of course, doctors who are trapped in the system and realize that they are part of the problem, but there are not too many "Patch Adams" out there. When you go to many doctors, they have one diagnosis for you: "Spend money, spend more money." That is basically it. The whole system is set up then to drain you and the insurance companies of your money.

Sounds like too terrible to believe, but that is what is happening to most patients. I am not saying I do not believe in the medical profession, by no means am I saying that. I think that there are times to take medication prescribed by a doctor. I think that there are times to have your bones put back together. I certainly do believe and understand the great science of surgery of the body, but oftentimes surgery is not the highest choice for healing. Sometimes some other method of treatment would be a better choice. The method or medication or herb or vegetable or fruit that may work with one person may not work as well with some other person. All of us humans are so different and so complex.

At this time we do not really have the intuitives on this planet in the medical profession who are needed to know and to work with patients on an individual basis. Ideally, an intuitive professional of medicine would spend an hour to two hours with each person, tuning into what that patient's needs are and then counseling with him or her about his or her health and what implementation is needed for healing. How wonderful this planet could be with that kind of medical care! That is what some who are aligned with Divine Administration will be trained for one day.

Energy Follows Thought

No food on this planet of dio decisions is really "pure." Even if foods are grown organically, there is the polluted air to consider, and, of course, the impurity of certain individuals who work with the food has to be considered—from the gardeners to the gatherers to the distributors to the cooks, and so on. Continuing Fifth

Epochal Revelation tells us that only in Divine Administration, where organic foods are being grown with the help of Celestial Overcontrol, are the foods beginning to be pure.

This is the same principle in any field; for example in midwifery if the midwife is technically correct but spiritually incorrect, what impact will she have on the mother and the baby? The Heisenberg theory indicates that each person looking through a microscope sees something different, based upon the individual's level of consciousness and frame of reference. Continuing Fifth Epochal Revelation expands upon this theory and states that this principle applies in all areas of reality. The consciousness of a person, where that person's soul is with God, changes what that person looks at, touches, etc. Matter responds to the thoughts, to the soul, to the spirit of persons.

It is important that people who want to heal, to get better, surround themselves with quality people, people who have their highest good in mind. And it is important that people who want to be healed adjust their thoughts to aid in their getting well.

The Necessity for Carefrontation in Ascension

Continuing Fifth Epochal Revelation teaches continued ascension. You cannot continue to be healed of your various maladies unless you continually ascend. With some diseases that you have manifested you have to ascend at an accelerated rate in order to be healed of them. You cannot jump on a bicycle; you have to jump into a Corvette, and some of you need to jump into a spaceship in order to reach your goal of overcoming the disease.

The word *carefrontation* is sometimes used as a synonym of *confrontation*. What a beautiful concept to understand—that a confrontation can truly be a carefrontation if it comes from someone who has your highest good in mind, especially genuine spiritual elders. When you can accept with grace and appreciation the admonishment and confrontation of people who love you and who are mature and who do not compromise with evil, you will be able to respond and change much more quickly. Carefrontation works beautifully as long as you can receive it and not get angry, not think that the carefronter dislikes you and is trying to hurt you. In Divine Administration carefrontation should always be done in love, not in resentment.

Some of you tend to hang onto anger, resentment, and guilt. You want to punish yourselves for your past mistakes and do not see yourselves forgiven by God. Divine Administration provides morontia counseling, which includes carefrontation and encouragement. Morontia counseling will be the reality continually through your sojourn on the mansion worlds after you pass on from this world, but it is beginning here on Urantia in Divine Administration.

Don't think, "Once I have passed onto the first mansion world, I am done with all that eldership stuff." It is only beginning, and the more you can ascend now on Urantia the more quickly you can pass through the first few mansion worlds. You will be able to visit those first few if you want, visit some friends that are on the first and second mansion worlds, but you might just skip to the third, to the fourth, to the fifth—hopping, skipping, and jumping through Satania. That is what Divine Administration here is being set up to do, to help you to hop, skip, and jump so that you can become administrators and teachers for others more quickly.

Paladin said that your thinking in the mansion worlds will more quickly manifest your thoughts in the "physical." Continuing Fifth Epochal Revelation states that wherever Divine Administration is manifested on Urantia will be the equivalent of a mansion world, depending upon the consciousness level of most of the people in that sector. So, those presently in Global Community Communications Alliance, who are experiencing Divine Administration being implemented on the beginning levels, are also experiencing in part the beginning mansion worlds. Be careful what you think and say, for you may manifest in the physical your dio as well as your Deo thoughts.

Persons in this world can have such physical beauty on the outside and be very ugly on the inside. As time goes on, however, that physical beauty diminishes. In my song "The Great American Dream" I wrote, "Miss America, your beauty is long gone." Usually outwardly pretty people who are not really good persons lose their physical beauty and begin to manifest in some way their inner ugliness, and often manifest sickness and die.

At the First Planetary Sacred Home many may get sicker more quickly with symptoms from what was manifested before aligning with Divine Administration. Many individuals are finding out the relationship of their minds and souls to their bodies, and they are discovering that the relationship is much more realized in Divine Administration; it manifests so much more quickly. If we receive carefrontation properly, we can begin to look so beautiful in our symptoms and begin to heal. We all have to flow with God through what is happening, each of us at our own level. What is Celestial Overcontrol asking of you?

The Healing Process Can Be Very Challenging

We all have our "cross to bear," as the Catholics say. Sometimes it gets very heavy, but never too heavy for us to carry with the help of Christ Michael, who can lighten it for us. The cross was very heavy for Jesus to carry at times, especially at the very end of His life. I like the idea of the spiritual lessons that can be learned in the thirteen Stations of the Cross. It is a beautiful, beautiful symbol of our spiritual ascension and growth.

When dealing with your brothers and sisters, do not expect them to be the same as you, though you may share similar experiences, especially with those in Divine Administration, which is a form of mansion world parallel. You need to be more patient with each other. The longer you practice this, the more you begin to notice that when you need lifting up, your brothers and sisters will lift you up. When you need to lift them up, you can lift them up. That is how it should work all over the world, but even more so in Divine Administration where moral and ethical standards are even higher, and those aligned have a deeper understanding of what each other is going through.

In Divine Administration especially, we begin to see glimpses of the actualization of our destinies. However, we are still living in our potentiality, not necessarily in actualization. We are told our destinies, and a lot of us begin to see it happening, see ourselves in the future. We get glimpses of our higher selves, of actually becoming what our higher cosmic names mean, of our higher realities.

Then we look in the mirror and become disappointed and manifest certain symptoms. “Oh my God, I am dying.” It is just symptoms you know, it is not really what is happening, really truly, but the symptoms. But all of a sudden you do not see yourself anymore in that destiny and the actualization of that destiny. You see yourself in some grave somewhere or in old age, not being able to manifest your destiny.

I constantly battle that myself; that is why I say I am twenty-nine eternally in my higher self because my lower self constantly wants to make me much older. But I do not let my body dictate to me what my lower self is trying to tell me. I have to be able to understand within my higher self what that lower self is, dealing with life on a fallen world. I am sure in many of my past lives that lower self won out. In some lives I allowed myself to get too depressed and overwrought by the many challenges in life, in spite of wonderful ideals and ideas I may have held. I know that in some of my past lives my arrogance led to my early death. I am sure that in some lives I trusted people when I should not have; maybe I had misplaced compassion that led me to the rack.

I had to learn what takes people off of this planet. I had to be taken off this planet many times with all those things to find out what it is. I learned to such a degree that if I allow myself right now to get into a state of fear I would freeze like an ice cube. I have to overcome all those fears from the deaths that I have gone through in past lives, and the diseases that I have had in past lives. I know that in one life as a gentle monk I died of disease because I got imbalanced in the Mother circuits. There was no reason for that to happen, but it happened. I allowed it to happen in my thinking processes, and the diseases took me. God does not go against His own laws. We manifest what we think. He has written the laws of cause and effect in time and eternity.

We do not have to be bound by disease and sickness; let us choose ascension and actualization. I desire to live by God’s laws. God help me to understand them. God help you to understand them. They are the laws we want to walk in. We cannot be stifled by our own errors or sinful natures. We cannot be stifled by the unwillingness of others to ascend at our willingness level. We cannot be stifled by that. When our mothers, fathers, sisters, brothers, or some of our friends do not want to ascend with us, then we need to grow without them. We need to ascend, regardless of what our loved ones decide. They will be with us always in eternity, and if not in this life, we will see them in the mansion worlds.

We find that even here at the First Planetary Sacred Home it is hard to eat healthy, natural, organic foods—vegetables and meat. So what are we doing? We are growing our own in the Third Garden of Eden. But it is not just those beautiful organic vegetables and fruits that are going to heal us; it is inner growth through correction and ascension.

I believe the greatest challenge that those at the First Planetary Sacred Home have is to wait for the perfection of God's perfect will for their unique destinies as Cosmic and Urantian Reservists. All of those aligned with Divine Administration have been chosen to try out to become a Cosmic or Urantian Reservist; that is why they are part of this great enterprise and experiment. They must wait; they must be patient for God's manifestation on this fallen world; they must wait for the rest of humanity's consciousness in their lower states to even begin to understand where those in Divine Administration are at.

What a challenge! They all want to be understood (as most humans do), and rightfully so. Those in Divine Administration know they have something more beautiful to give the world. They have epochal revelation and continuing epochal revelation. They have the synthesis of the totality of all that has gone on in the history of this planet now conceptualized, captured here in the truth and teachings of Continuing Fifth Epochal Revelation.

The potentials for those in Divine Administration are like a bottle with a wonderful little genie in it that is thrown out into the ocean of truth, beauty, and goodness. But boy can that bottle be hard to find! So, patience, patience, patience, patience. I had been thinking that my destiny was going to be completely fulfilled a long time ago. I had my own ideas about how this would happen, and my destiny is partially fulfilled, but not completely, and not always in the way I thought it would happen.

Within Divine Administration it is more difficult for Niánn and me, and the difficulty lessens from the higher Eldership mandates down through the other mandate levels to students, some of whom one day can themselves become Elders. It is difficult for us to be patient in waiting for the manifestation of the Divine New Order of the future; we are only living in such a small aspect of the Divine New Order ourselves, a very small aspect.

I wanted some of my dreams to happen with my first album, a vinyl album that I did for God in 1985. I thought it was going to happen then, and I was kind of angry at God because it did not happen then. I did everything that I thought I could do right; I thought I was ready. I had *The URANTIA Book*. I had God, and I had the music. But what I did not have was Continuing Fifth Epochal Revelation.

I really did not know who the heck I was. I had no idea of who I was in past lives. I had no idea that I would be an audio fusion material complement. I had no idea that I was supposed to bring Continuing Fifth Epochal Revelation to the world. I just thought, "I have *The URANTIA Book*; I have this spiritual music; the world needs it, and the world needs it right now." I was so upset when God thought differently. And so what happened? I got sick. I manifested different symptoms, and I was in depression for months and months at a time. So, for whatever reason that your destiny is on hold, the time lag of justice may seem like an eternity to you.

It is so easy to lose faith in your vision. Concerning the time lag of justice, in *The URANTIA Book* on page 616 it says:

> Supreme justice can act instantly when not restrained by divine mercy. But the ministry of mercy to the children of time and space always provides for this time lag, this saving interval between seedtime and harvest. If the seed sowing is good, this interval provides for the testing and upbuilding of character; if the seed sowing is evil, this merciful delay provides time for repentance and rectification. This time delay in the adjudication and execution of evildoers is inherent in the mercy ministry of the seven superuniverses. This restraint of justice by mercy proves that God is love, and that such a God of love dominates the universes and in mercy controls the fate and judgment of all his creatures.

We must not lose sight of who we are as *ascending* sons and daughters of God. None of us who are aspiring for true healing can lose sight.

We must persevere throughout the trials and learn to "fatten" on those disappointments. Your healing is within you and within your relationship to God—your connection to the healing, to the divine, to the ascension, to the destiny, to the actualization, to the service of humankind—that is your healing.

The Healing of the Body or The Whitewashing of the Soul; Healing and Moving into Point-of-Origin Reconstruction

by Gabriel of Urantia and Niánn Emerson Chase

Teaching by Niánn Emerson Chase

Why is it that some people who make a commitment to be on a serious spiritual path seem to suddenly feel much better, and others suddenly begin to feel aches and pains? It seems to be a discrepancy, but it is not. Continuing Fifth Epochal Revelation states that the system of Satania is presently in the adjudication of Lucifer versus Gabriel of Salvington. It is also the adjudication of this planet and of each individual on Urantia.

Different things happen for different people, and there are different manifestations within our individual spiritual ascension, our personal adjudication, reconciliation, and healing processes. It is very important that we do not go around judging someone else because, "I am feeling on top of the world, and this person is not, so they are more dio than I am." That may not be the case at all. Healing and growth are strictly individualistic; we are all complex human beings.

A *fourth-dimensional physician*—who knows and applies the truths in *The URANTIA Book* and Continuing Fifth Epochal Revelation ascension science, and who deals with the physical body and the mind and soul—will tell you that just on the physical level, people are such individuals that their healing processes are quite different. Physicians in the third dimension—doctors who deal only with physical symptoms in their patients without the higher understanding of the psychospiritual variables, who are the majority of doctors—will tell you that what works for one person may not work for the next person who has the same so-called disease or illness. Why is that?

Some are aware from common sense, as well as from the epochal revelation found in *The URANTIA Book* and *The Cosmic Family* volumes, that there are illnesses and physical ailments that are due to outside influences—our genetics, the environment, and accidents. Some know that many aspects of the environment are very toxic now due to human-caused pollution of air, soil, water, plants, and animals; this pollution can cause many health problems. There are a lot of viruses and harmful bacteria that may impact our health. It may be that for one person who is impacted by a virus, that illness is a spiritual lesson for him or her, but for the person next to him or her, who also is ill from the virus, the sickness has nothing to do with anything spiritual at all. Health (good or bad) is a very individualized thing. Most people are not at the ascension level of spiritual insight to discern why someone else is physically ill. That is what judgment is about, and most people are not in a place to judge anyone.

There are illnesses that have to do with a person's inner status, his or her rebellion and lack of adherence to some of God's laws. We know for fourth-order starseed, as well as for many Urantians, that incorrect thought, which Continuing Fifth Epochal Revelation refers to as dio thought, can, and has, led to rebellion, which then can be the cause of our physical discomforts.

Rebellion is a Cancer

Rebellion is a cancer for many of us, and some are more infected than others. Cancer, as we all know, is an unhealthy state wherein certain cells begin to specialize; they "self-assert" themselves and no longer work in union or synchronization with the rest of the body system, like secession from divine administration. (On that small cellular level, you can see how cancer is like the Lucifer Rebellion.) Self-assertion happens within the cells, and that is what creates cancer and other problems. If those dio cells, those cancer cells specializing in self-assertion, continue, they create an ugly tumor, and that tumor, if the cells continue this, will grow and spread.

Many of us have lost a loved one to cancer, and we know what it did to the body of our beloved one. The cancer just spread and grew. One system after another began to malfunction until that cancer permeated every aspect of the body, so that there eventually was a complete shutdown.

It is the same thing as when individuals begin to make choices in their self-assertion, and if they continue making those choices they are creating that cancer within themselves and in their consciousness. It is then that it becomes a sin, and if they continue in that, it grows and permeates them and then develops into iniquity and will eventually cause the shutdown of that individual if he or she chooses to continue in that. Annihilation then can happen unless that is reverted.

The great spiritual physicians are about attempting to help people reverse that cancerous rebellion within them. According to Continuing Fifth Epochal Revelation, the remission and healing of cancer begins when those dio cells stop actualizing in self-assertion and revert back to a healthy state and being. In the medical field, some physicians are aware of certain patients whose cancer cells all of a sudden stop asserting themselves and start reverting back to what they were supposed to be in divine pattern, and most of these doctors have no understanding of why this remission happens. Why does remission happen for some people and not others? It is so important in the healing process that these cells go back into that healthy state. When they do, they are no longer in self-assertion; they return to interdependency, to union, and synchronization with the rest of the systems of the body so that they again have a "sense" of responsibility for each other.

When you choose to move into Luciferic self-assertion, you move away from feeling that sense of cosmic obligation to others, just like cancer cells do. In order to revert back into your healthy state, your point-of-origin reconstruction, you have to go into realizing who you really are and move back to that union of souls. Starseed and Urantians need to do that, to reverse dio patterns and self-assertion. In their evaluation of themselves in Global Community Communications Alliance, individuals are beginning to see their harmful patterns and are working at reversing these patterns; they are working at healing themselves. Starseed want to go back to their "point-of-origin reconstruction," and Urantians want to go back into divine pattern, back into perfect "personality circuitry," back into their own "individual personality pattern."

That is the meaning of healing, when you can begin to evaluate yourself and choose then to go back to what you really were and who you really are so that you can move forward again. Rebellion is stopping you, pulling you off a path of rightness, a path of evolution and ascension. Before you can move forward again, you have to go back to where you were pulled off, thus the concept "back to point-of-origin reconstruction" or back to where you were in your rightness at whatever level. That is what the first and second mansion worlds are all about, getting you there, getting rid of all of those discrepancies and problems that you have so that you can start moving forward again.

In a previous teaching I pointed out that *Merriam Webster's Collegiate Dictionary* defines healing as, "making sound or whole; restoring to health, mending; overcoming; patching up a breach or division; restoring to original purity or integrity." Those beautiful definitions take on even newer meaning for all who are seeking truth, reconciliation, and healing. According to Fifth Epochal Revelation, real healing is *an organized dissolution of chaos*, because being out of God's will is chaos. Pulling away from the unity and the unification that is found in divine pattern does create disunity, brokenness, and chaos.

I think most people have felt "chaotic"—some more regularly than others. Rebellion is first and foremost pulling away from the Universal Father, and when you do that, it is just downhill from then on, pulling away from everything that is good and pure and whole, and as you do that, you become more and more disunified, dysfunctional. As you pull away from the representatives of the Universal Father—the Creator Sons, the various ministering spirits, and the teachers that are sent—you become even more and more dysfunctional, and it will eventually result in a physical illness because your body then lacks physical unification within it. There is a brokenness that happens in the systems in your body that will physically manifest the disunification that is happening within you, between the emerging soul and the spirit of God.

Our whole living energy system (body, mind, and soul) has to get out of that brokenness and become unified in order for us to heal. What is our unifier? It is the personality, and that is why Continuing Fifth Epochal Revelation, especially in *The Cosmic Family, Volume II*, puts so much emphasis on the importance of moving into personality pattern, of moving into personality circuitry.

One paper uses the word "personality" twenty-eight times in its five pages. There is just so much emphasis on being within the personality circuitry from the Universal Father. We have to relinquish our "self-made identities" in order to move into our real "God-pattern identities," which are found in our personality, our personality circuitry. Our self-made identity is chaos. It has to dissolve, and that can be very painful.

> . . . the concept of the personality as the meaning of the whole of the living and functioning [not malfunctioning] creature means much more than the integration of relationships; it signifies the *unification* of all factors of reality as well as coordination of relationships. Relationships exist between two objects, but three or more objects eventuate a *system,* and such a system is much more than just an enlarged or complex relationship. [Think of that system within your bodies, on a microscopic level, but think of it too in divine administration on a cosmic level, because it goes all the way. The word *system* is used on all levels.] This distinction is vital, for in a cosmic system the individual members are not connected with each other except in relation to the whole and through the individuality of the whole. (*The URANTIA Book,* p. 1227)

Lucifer pulled everyone away from the system, pulled them away from the idea of the whole. That is what self-assertion is all about. Self-assertion is self-absorption. Remember the difference between self-absorption and self-evaluation? It is walking that beautiful line, being a unique individual, and realizing that we have our individual processes, but in our individuality we are interconnected with each other. It is being able to be an individual and yet be part of a whole and feel that corporate connection.

At the First Planetary Sacred Home, the healing department is called, "The Council on *Unified* Health and Life Services," for the importance of unification within God's will and His pattern is realized. The emphasis is first with the inner status of the ailing individual, for it is understood that the inner state is very often the cause of the physical status. What is happening inside psychologically and spiritually, *psychospiritually*, is usually going to be the cause of your physical status, especially in Divine Administration. Those in Global Community Communications Alliance are called to first and foremost become ministers and teachers, bringing the Fifth and Continuing Fifth Epochal Revelation to others, for it is that higher truth, lodged in individual minds, that will bring their true healing.

Spiritual Priorities in the Healing Process

Just as Michael of Nebadon was instructed by Immanuel before bestowing on Urantia as Jesus, Gabriel of Urantia and I too have been instructed by Michael in our mandate on Urantia to "give attention first to the liberation and inspiration of man's spiritual nature." These are our priorities in our ministry. Give attention, *first*, to the liberation and inspiration of humans' spiritual nature. *Next*, illuminate the darkened human intellect, heal the souls of men, and emancipate their minds from age-old fears. And *then*, in accordance with our mortal wisdom, minister to the physical well-being and material comfort of our brothers and sisters in the flesh. These instructions are found in *The URANTIA Book* on page 1328 in the second paragraph.

The ministry of Global Community Communications Alliance first addresses the spiritual nature of an individual, then the psychological (intellectual and emotional), then the physical. That is why Divine Administration's main outreach to the world at this time is disseminating the truths of epochal revelation, whether the dissemination comes through classes offered in schools; books and other printed materials; teachings on audio cassettes, videos, CDs, and DVDs; art presented by artists; plays performed by adult and children dramatists; or music presented by choirs and bands.

Because this is the adjudication, it is even more important for people to take care of their inner business. In each person's adjudication this means reconciliation with God and unification of your being. Then healing can happen. You first have to reconcile with your God before you can begin to unify all of your systems for actual healing to begin.

As was emphasized, each one is treated individually in this adjudication, in this reconciliation, unification, and healing process. What it takes for one person to come into restoration of his or her entire system is going to be different for another. For many, that "organized dissolution of your chaos" means first being physically ill before you can move into unification. In order for your physical body to be restored to its point-of-origin reconstruction or correct personality circuitry, your consciousness needs to be adjusted, which can create tremendous conflict in your psychospiritual body as well as in your physical one.

You probably have experienced a tremendous inner conflict that happens when your thought processes are challenged, your belief systems are challenged, your mind is stretched, and you are asked to go even further in your attainment of truth and virtue. For those aligned in Divine Administration, they are asked every day to keep going further and further in their ascension. (Actually, the Spirit of God is asking this of everyone on this world, but most are fleeing from that Voice or have shut It out completely.) For those at the First Planetary Sacred Home that Voice is not going to stop, and there is tremendous conflict, and often psychospiritual conflict will manifest physically too. Physical symptoms manifest—aching stomachs, terrible headaches, achy bones, and so forth—all due to the conflict that an individual is struggling with and dealing with in his or her own personal adjudication and healing process.

In Divine Administration, the higher the mandate the higher the responsibility, and the greater the conflict that can happen before restoration. What some are discovering is that the processes that they go through inwardly on psychological and spiritual levels can manifest simultaneously within their bodies.

Continuing Fifth Epochal Revelation discusses (in one of the many community transmissions) "instant karma" on another world in the universe of Avalon. On that world, if there was a deviation from God's plan within the mind of a person, that deviation instantly manifested physically in him or her. Those physical manifestations of disease can in reality be a blessing if we listen to what our body and the spirit of God is communicating to us, for the physical symptoms can be signs to show the way to our inner problems that need to be addressed.

When sensitive and tender persons grieve over the state of the planet, they can manifest that grief physically too. They feel much compassion for the suffering and sometimes a sense of helplessness that they cannot just stop all of this pain, especially when they think of children and how they are used and exploited. That gets to me more than anything else, the suffering of children. Reports of the hundreds of thousands, even millions, of children who are being abused and exploited really tear me up.

Continuing Fifth Epochal Revelation has stated that if you do not feel grief at times over the state of the planet, then you have not moved to that place of God's compassion that you need to. We can feel joy; we can be cheerful and rejoice in the wonderful blessings in our lives, and at the same time, we can be filled with a tremendous grief and sorrow at the suffering that is happening to so many of our brothers and sisters all over the world. But we cannot be crippled or debilitated by our grief over the suffering of so many. Much of our healing is learning how to deal with the frustration, grief, and sorrow that comes from our compassion for others' struggling and suffering. Much of our healing includes *acting,* becoming *activists*, as a result of those emotions.

The Phenomenon of Mass Healing

Miraculous healings can happen and have happened on Urantia. One of the largest was with Jesus when almost seven hundred people were spontaneously healed, and Jesus was saying, "What happened here?". He had had a big day with His apostles, and they had gone to the Zebedee house. It was a big house where He and His apostles often gathered. That night, Perpetua, Peter's wife (who usually did the cooking for Jesus, the apostles, and other disciples who gathered together), heard a racket outside and went out to look.

There were hundreds of people outside the house, and Perpetua said, "Master, I have a problem outside here. I cannot feed all these people. They are clamoring for you." When Jesus went out to look at them He saw mostly the sick people who were asking for help. They had heard about this wonderful teacher and healer, and they had come to Him. What happened is that Jesus looked upon them with His compassion, and spontaneously they were all healed. It was one of the largest of what we would call genuine miraculous healings that has ever happened on the planet. There were six hundred and eighty-three men, women, and children whose physical ailments were instantly gone.

> The sight of these afflicted mortals, men, women, and children, suffering in large measure as a result of the mistakes and misdeeds of His own trusted Sons of universe administration, peculiarly touched the human heart of Jesus and challenged the divine mercy of this benevolent Creator Son.

You can find the detailed description of this episode on pages 1632 and 1633 in *The URANTIA Book*. I highly recommend that you read it.

Miraculous healings have happened since that time in the Zebedee yard two thousand years ago. These kinds of healings of individuals and groups of individuals, these spontaneous, miraculous healings of physical illness, usually happen with people whose physical symptoms are caused more by the outer state of affairs rather than by their inner state.

This happened at other times in Jesus' ministry too. On page 1669, beginning with the first paragraph, to the top of 1670, *The URANTIA Book* discusses "spontaneous" and "unconscious healing." (I highly recommend that you read that on your own.) Those in Divine Administration believe that this kind of spontaneous and mass healing is going to happen for certain individuals at the Sacred Concerts when The Bright and Morning Star Band plays. We also are aware that this kind of physical healing cannot remain with those people unless a spiritual change point personally happens for them.

Going back to Jesus' healing of the 683 people, we are told in *The URANTIA Book* about those people:

> But the majority of those who were recipients of supernatural or creative physical healing at this sundown demonstration of divine energy were not permanently spiritually benefited by this extraordinary manifestation of mercy. A small number were truly edified by the physical ministry, but the spiritual kingdom was not advanced in the hearts of [persons] by this amazing eruption of timeless creative healing.

So, it was a temporary state of affairs for the majority of those people; for most of them nothing really spiritual happened. No spiritually meaningful change point happened to them. Recall what Immanuel's instructions were to Michael before He came to the planet as Jesus—that He should take care first of the spiritual status of the people, then their minds, and then He could deal with the physical.

Repentance and Healing

In order for a lasting healing to happen, an individual must be willing to repent. Because fourth-order starseed have somehow pulled away from God, they must be willing to repent and then revert back to God. I want to mention two examples of people at the First Planetary Sacred Home who, when aligning with Divine Administration, right away started healing their physical ailments, and the reason they did is because there had been a shift in their minds.

For one middle-aged, starseed *URANTIA Book* reader, the shift process began to happen to her before she actually was even aware of Divine Administration. She had already acquiesced that she wanted to reconcile with God. She began to do that, and a few months later, she discovered the Continuing Fifth Epochal Revelation and immediately responded to it and aligned with Global Community Communications Alliance. Within months her physical ailments were gone.

An elderly first-time Urantian woman (a new soul) who had some physical problems before she moved to the community and began her spiritual path, began getting more and more youthful once she embraced the process of truth and reconciliation that is part of the everyday life in Global Community Communications Alliance. Her energy is much higher now, and many of her symptoms have abated or lessened. For others there was already a shift beginning to happen before coming to the community, and the healing has continued to happen.

Healing is a long, life-long process (actually for some lives-long), and you must continually be open and receptive to the admonishment of God. For you starseed, you are still in the process of repenting and in the process of reverting back to what God wants you to be in your point-of-origin reconstruction. For new souls, you are repenting and progressing into your new construction within God's blueprint for you.

There is a lot of wonderful information in Continuing Fifth Epochal Revelation on tron therapy, and a lot of that comes out in *The Cosmic Family*, *Volume II*, and even more in *Volume III*. It can bring an instant, spontaneous healing of the physical body only if that individual who is receiving this therapy is repentant; that is a prerequisite, being truly repentant and then willing to bring a change point into his or her consciousness and to continue on that path, to continue moving forward, to continue bringing those change points.

The fact is that healing really must happen in the mind and soul first before it can manifest in the body. Remember, *The URANTIA Book* says "energy follows thought." As our thoughts are transformed, our bodies will be transformed. I want to close with some words that Jesus gave to those who loved and followed Him. He said:

> Seek the greater thing, and the lesser will be found therein; ask for the heavenly, and the earthly shall be included. The shadow is certain to follow the substance. (*The URANTIA Book,* p. 1823)

We know that the substance, the reality, is in your soul. Your body is just the shadow, the temporary, and so it has to happen first in the soul, in your spirit. Seek that first, that healing, and then the shadow (the body) is sure to follow.

I would like to remind everyone of the title of this teaching, "The Healing of the Body or The Whitewashing of the Soul; Healing and Moving into Point-of-Origin Reconstruction."

Nourishing the soul can bring healing to the body. The soul is something that needs nourishment in order to grow and expand. Do you feed your soul? What do you feed your soul? I caution people out there working in the third dimension (mainstream society) to watch what they feed their souls, because that is going to indicate how healthy their body is going to be and stay. Those in Global Community Communications Alliance constantly try to reprogram themselves to come out of the third-dimensional materialistic values and into the fourth-dimensional values of compassion and spiritual truths. Fourth-dimensional thinking, feeling, and doing will feed our souls so that we can gain, as Niánn said, our "God-given identities."

Images

What is your image of the world? What image do you have of yourself? Some of your images are like a tiny ant or like a tiny insect. Some of your images are like a turtle. Now a turtle could be good. Usually when you think of a turtle you think of it moving very slowly and methodically through life. Sometimes I am like a turtle where I go very cautiously and slowly, looking around, making sure that everything is OK. Then, I go inside the shell and think about the situation for a while longer before I take a first step.

You could be like an eagle; you could feel like an eagle, rising high above the daily mundane circumstances in order to have an expanded perception. You can feel like a road-runner nervously running in many directions or a lion ready to growl at the first sign of someone not in agreement with you. You could be like a wise owl. You could be like a donkey, so stubborn you will never move; you do not care if somebody is right, you are just not going to move.

So we have all these animal identifications, and we all have different aspects of those animal tendencies in us. We are of animal origin, but in being human we have to come above the animal natures and incorporate the good tendencies in all those animals to help us become higher human mortals.

Building a Body Instrument for Serving the Planet

You could also identify yourselves with a big skyscraper, standing isolated with its gleaming glass beaming. It can appear to be so fragile that if a great wind came along the building might blow right over, and yet in reality be resilient and able to withstand great earthquakes and strong winds. It can also look very strong, firm, and beautiful on the outside, but the inside may be empty. The skyscraper may have a lot of glitter on the outside, but it is all superficial if the inside is like a vacuum and has no inner life.

You can be another kind of building. You can be like the buildings that incorporate sacred architecture and divine principles of usage. You know that whatever is happening inside of that building is not just for appearance but for the sake of what is outside of the building: the world. That building, that body, is not just serving itself; that building, that body, is serving the planet. Your body is your building, lovely to behold—alive, breathing, part of nature, part of God—and you just know that whatever is happening inside, it is serving the world.

Are you one with God? Because being one with God makes you an instrument for service in His name. He has built you to serve the world. For example, the individuals of Global Community Communications Alliance think of themselves as world souls, not just individual souls, but as world servers. Alice Bailey used the terms "world servers" and "world souls" in her teachings by Djwal Khul.

You just know that your building is built not just for you, not just for one person, and not for one group but for the world, the entire planet. That is why you are here on this planet. That is why

God created you, giving you existence so that you can become a world server, a planet server, a system server.

Those of Global Community Communications Alliance often end their prayers with this phrase: "for the common good of all in the system of Satania." Why did God build you? Well, He made you for the system of Satania; He made you for the universe of Nebadon, for the superuniverse that you are living in; He made you for the master universe, with you eventually becoming a finaliter. Throughout your ascension in eternity, you continue to serve. That is what finality is, eternal service. That is what being healthy is.

As you grow, you serve. Are you more in service to others? As you become more in service to others your soul becomes interlinked to a universal lifeline. Did you ever hear of a universal soul? Your existence becomes part of the breathing mechanism of the whole planet. *The URANTIA Book* says that the grand universe, with Paradise at its center, breathes in and out. Why does it do that? I think because it is the center of the soul of everything else, and as you breathe with it, it is created for everything else, and you are created for everything else. It is all one for the good of the whole.

The ultimate goal for any work is service for the people of the planet. If work is just for paying the rent, paying the bills with no sense of higher purpose or meaning, then it is just a job, not meaningful work. If your work is just for yourself and you feel that you are burdened to provide for yourself all on your own, you need to come to a higher understanding of meaningful work.

Some of you have not learned to step aside and realize that God supports you. Many people have not even learned that lesson yet. Many are still trying to support themselves, and that is why they basically struggle in supporting themselves, because they have not learned yet that they should be serving others. That is why when someone has ripped you off five or ten dollars, you are so mad at them you want to break their neck. What? Five or ten bucks, a thousand bucks, ten thousand dollars—what is a friendship worth with somebody? What kind of price do you put on a person? Does money mean more to you than the soul who is sitting or standing next to you?

Where does your worth lie? Do not wait for love to come to you. Go out and love. Be love. Do not wait to be given to, but give to others. Give. The reason why most of the people are miserable in this world is that they have never learned those two things—allowing God in their lives and serving others—they are still wanting what they want just for themselves. They are self-absorbed, the center of their own universe; everything revolves around them. Your existence, your talents, everything that you "are" should be for the world, to bring God to the world in some way through every talent that you have. Your work in some way should manifest the magnificence, the beauty, the dignity, the goodness, the love of God to someone else.

Your soul is like a mountain spring. Did you ever look at a creek and wonder about the water? That water just keeps coming, and every drop becomes a part of other drops to form the creek, which eventually joins a river, the river then joining other rivers to eventually become part of the ocean. Each drop of water is significant. Each of you is as a drop of water and significant. Each one of you is part of the ocean of God.

Each one of you is a different building in the holy city of God. The physical building right now houses your soul. Your soul is what is important; your soul is the true mechanism.

Those aligned with Divine Administration are beginning to learn corporate thinking. Niánn was teaching about "corporate understanding," "community consciousness," and "divine administration." The whole becomes more important now than just the individual self. Those individuals evolving into more of a community consciousness, a corporate understanding, outgrow thinking of himself or herself as the greatest; they think of themselves as part of something that is great, part of a team that is great, part of a divine administration that serves all.

Those in Divine Administration are trying to get there, trying to understand how that works. When any one complains because he or she has to dig a ditch or do something else that he or she feels is below them, in those instances that person is not being a significant water drop that is part of the whole. It does not matter what kind of work you do within God's will; what is more important is what God needs you to do as His mortal instrument. I learn this more and more all the time.

Is God the Father of Your Moments?

Administration is like a wheel, it does not matter what office you are in, what position you are in, you are part of the wheel, and every part is significant, no matter the function. Divine administration is a wheel within the master universe. You become part of that continual movement; nothing is more important than anything else; all of you working in divine pattern are significant. We just have different functions. Sometimes, you may want to be over here or over there, but God wants you to be of higher service in another area.

As I began to walk more consciously and more closely with God—not only in this life but also in many others—a lot of my moments were not the moments that I wanted to spend. If it would have been up to just me, my moment, I would have been doing something else, and when I got out of God's perfect will into His permissive will, I was into my moments but not into God's moments, and so my body got sicker. In some way, I was not functioning; my body was not responding, so I had aches and pains and this and that. We can have those aches and pains for many reasons, but here I am talking specifically about being out of the will of God and causing our own misery. There is enough misery that comes our way, even when we are in the perfect will of God on a rebellious world. So do not help the cause of Caligastia (who some may understand to be the devil).

Consider a termite. It is very, very small. A termite alone is not much, one little termite, but you put a whole lot of them together and termites can build the biggest skyscraper in the world in relation to their size. These termites build magnificent structures. They get really excited when a couple of termites see other termites beginning to build, . . . sniff, sniff, . . . man, they sense each other and get excited! Pretty soon they are helping the other termites. They know exactly what to do.

If they are building this little thing over here, the termites then know exactly what to get to help build it on the other side. They are little architects, and pretty soon that termite mound gets bigger and bigger, eventually getting to the size of a tree. Little termites built it. There are different kinds of termites, and some of the termite mounds are six feet high or more.

That termite cooperation is similar to auhter energy between human beings building a higher reality. That is what God is trying to create in a divine administration. We all become important because of the corporate work we do as a team. We get the job done. We get it done in a magnificent way, and everyone benefits. One termite alone could not build that mound. One termite might be more capable than most others. One termite might be bigger or stronger than the majority. One termite might be smarter than most, but no matter how big the termite is or how smart, it does not have what it takes to build that big mound six feet tall by itself; it needs help. All those termites corporately understand that they need each other, and that is what makes the mound grow. God has made us humans the same way.

Know your limitations; know what you can do; know what you cannot do; know what you want to do but need training to do. Do not try to be something you are not. Accept what you are; accept what you are not. Trying to find that balance within yourself is not an easy task for many on Urantia, particularly when we are taught that we are supposed to be something we are not. Everyone is supposed to look like the person on TV and so on and so on, and we can get lost when trying to find our God-identity.

What is your image? What is your God-identity? Once you begin to find your God-identity in the personality of God, then the beauty and the magnificence of God comes out of you and you are more functional for God. Being used as an instrument of God does not mean that you have to be an administrator, because you might be more functional tomorrow in the garden swinging an ax. Do not think you are self-important because you are in an administrative office or working as a high-level manager. Do not think yourself more important because that is not the way the wheel of God works.

Be part of the band of God. What is a *band*? Look at it like a chain with all these links interconnected, banded together. All those different instruments banded together make it work, but one alone does not make it work. I never enjoyed myself just singing. I did to some degree, but I have always heard all these orchestrations. I have always heard all these musical instruments. I was never quite happy or complete just sitting and playing by myself, although I have been encouraged to, and at times it is OK, but I would sure like to be complemented by the bands of God, by the instruments of God.

So, we need to learn to play different instruments. You cannot just be in administration. Take a day off; go work on the land; use your instrument differently. Be open enough to hear from God, and you will be surprised what He may tell you to do. But if your importance is in that pencil and paper or that computer or in your title, then you need to evaluate yourself a little better because who you are is not what you do. I wrote the song, "It is not who you are but what is inside you." It is not the outside of the building; it is the inside, in the soul. So learn to play different instruments, for as you become more diversified and expanded, healing is a greater possibility for you.

Helping Each Other Grow and Heal

The healing has to come from increased consciousness, and you have to see what the bigger picture is. Some of you starseed, particularly, have problems that go back thousands and thousands and thousands of years, and it is not that easy just to touch you and be healed. It does not work like that. Within Divine Administration, trying to open up those circuits of understanding is my job. That is Niánn's job. That is the Elders' jobs, and the Elders are just beginning to understand. Opening up those circuits so that individuals can be healed is not an easy task because the Elders have not even completely opened their own circuits. Now the Eldership is beginning to get stronger, more solid, with a greater foundation. They are becoming more "cosmictized." Becoming more cosmictized enables a person to move on a little faster, at a greater rate, even though at times it may look like nothing is happening, but it is. It is happening.

ABBREVIATED GLOSSARY

of terms introduced and/or expanded upon in
The URANTIA Book or Continuing Fifth Epochal Revelation

* = terms introduced in Continuing Fifth Epochal Revelation or given a completely new meaning in Continuing Fifth Epochal Revelation

A

adjudication, the — the adjudication of the Lucifer Rebellion; administered by the Bright and Morning Star versus Lucifer in our local universe of Nebadon. Began in 1911 and continuing. Sometimes referred to as the "end times" or "apocalypse."

agondonter — an evolutionary mortal who can believe in spiritual things without seeing proof

ascension science* — fusion of science with spirit (or spirituality); interrelationship between scientific and spiritual aspects; includes the physics of rebellion

astral body* — a tangible entity (more spirit than physical)—but not exactly a "body" in the manner that human mortals may think of—that represents the circuitry of an individual personality's various past lives and encompasses that soul's memories and experiences that make up the personality's unique identity. A person's physical body can manifest certain aspects of his or her astral bodies because as an individual grows spiritually, he or she literally begins to change physically the look and form of the human body.

audio fusion material complement* — a fusion of a celestial personality with a mortal in the complete aonic to cellular reality of the lower being. The fusion takes place within the particle reality of the life force of the existing soul. On Urantia, Gabriel of Urantia is the only audio fusion material complement, used in bringing through continuing epochal revelation.

auhter energy* — a measurable energy field, created by souls in a cosmically related group of people

Avalon — a nearby local universe, including the area earth astronomers denominate the Pleiades

B

Bright and Morning Star, the — Gabriel of Salvington, the head administrative celestial being in our local universe; first-born son of Christ Michael and the Universe Mother Spirit

C

Caligastia — a celestial personality (Secondary Lanonandek Son) resident on Earth/Urantia who fell in the Lucifer Rebellion, at the time as the Planetary Prince of Urantia. He is sometimes referred to as "the devil" and has a legion of rebel forces working under him to create chaos and perpetrate evil and iniquity worldwide.

causal body* — the higher blueprint given at the beginning of a soul's birth into his or her first mother. On a fallen world, such as this one, the causal body should act as a guide, a higher chart, a diagram for intuitive counselors and medical doctors because the present emotional, astral, and physical bodies are far from the original design of the Creator.

Celestial Overcontrol* — celestial beings who help administer world affairs through a spiritual hierarchy in other dimensions

change point* — a time of purification; end times; transition from one spiritual dimension to another

Christ Michael — celestial ruler (Creator Son) of our local universe of Nebadon; incarnated as Jesus, Son of God

complements* — high spiritual mates; sometimes considered "soul mates". Spiritual complements can be pairs of male/female or 2 of same gender (but same gender pairs would never be sexual mates, only spiritual complements in work functions together).

Continuing Fifth Epochal Revelation* — the continuation of the Fifth Epochal Revelation (*The URANTIA Book*), much of which is available in *The Cosmic Family* volumes, transmitted through the Audio Fusion Material Complement Gabriel of Urantia. These teachings explain the physics of rebellion and ascension science, addressing the current state of the world and identifying the changes needed, on both individual and corporate levels, to truly solve planetary crises.

cosmic circles — *See* psychic circles

cosmic family* — cosmically-connected, genetically-related souls; often from past lives on this planet and/or other worlds

Cosmic Reservist* — starseed human mortals assigned and trained to aid in times of planetary emergency, particularly spiritual crises; a.k.a. change agents.

Creator Son — the Universe Father of a local universe, celestial personality who co-rules a local universe with a Creative Daughter/Universe Mother Spirit as complements to each other. In Nebadon, Jesus Christ Michael is the Creator Son who rules as our Universe Sovereign.

D

Deo* — good; godly; of God

Deo-particle energy* — atomic and sub-atomic energy in divine pattern

Deo thade thought patterns* — acting on a series of thoughts based on godly and good foundations

Destiny Reservist — human mortals assigned and trained to aid in times of planetary emergency, particularly spiritual crises; a.k.a. change agents. *See also* Cosmic and Urantian Reservists.
dio* — bad; evil; ungodly; not of God
dio cells* — cells out of divine pattern, created by wrong attitudes and behavior in an individual
dio thade thought patterns* — acting on a series of erroneous and harmful thoughts
diotribes* — negative or harmful particles in the body, caused by thoughts outside of divine pattern
Divine Administration* — a hierarchy of spiritual leaders (human mortals and celestials) mandated to assist with the solving of world affairs

E

energy reflective circuit* — vortexes (vortices) of energy; power spots around the planet; used for celestial transport and communication
epochal revelation — worldwide prophetic knowledge (revelation) about God and the cosmos, given to the planet by celestial personalities at periodic intervals. On Earth/Urantia there have been 5 epochal revelations.
etheric body (emotional body)* — the body between the physical and the astral, sometimes called the emotional body, but it is related to the morontia body of the ovan soul
evolutionary religion — the various religions of the world that evolved throughout history from human perceptions and ideas about God, other celestial personalities, and the cosmos and containing both some truths and falsehoods. Evolutionary religions are in contrast to revelatory religion (information given by God and celestial personalities directly to mortals).

F

famotor* — movement and form of the body based on spiritual realities; visually recognizable reflection of the soul within the body
Father-circuited* — representing the qualities of the Universe Father, much like a human father, in responses: strong, decisive, leading, protecting, guiding, etc.
Fifth Epochal Revelation — revelatory information published as *The URANTIA Book* and containing more than 2,000 pages of facts about God, the cosmos, and many of the celestial and mortal inhabitants of the grand universe. *The URANTIA Book* was first printed in 1955, although the information contained therein came to the planet beginning in the 1930s.
finaliter — highly ascended, old soul (once a mortal but now a celestial personality) who has attained "finality" in the ascension to Paradise
first-light soul* — new soul in his or her first mortal life

First Planetary Sacred Home, the* — spiritual administrative center of a planet; Planetary Headquarters; the location changes as a gathering place for spiritual renaissances throughout history
first stage of light and life — the first of seven successive stages of an inhabited, evolutionary world becoming progressively more settled in spiritual attainments and refined existence levels reflecting divine pattern in all ways
first-time Urantian* — new/first-light soul whose native planet of origin is Urantia (Earth); a soul who has had no previous lives
fourth dimension* — the next dimension that is higher on a consciousness level as well on a "material" level, that of morontia
fourth-order starseed* — persons who have had past lives on other worlds in other universes and who participated in some manner in rebellion against God's laws
fruits of the spirit — spiritual qualities such as love, joy, peace, long-suffering, gentleness, goodness, faith, meekness, and temperance

G

Gabriel of Salvington — *See* the Bright and Morning Star
Garden of Eden — on Urantia, the First Garden of Eden was started by Van and Amadon in preparation for Adam and Eve about 38,000 years ago. (That site is now submerged under the Mediterranean Sea.) After their default, Adam and Eve left the "First Garden" and established a Second Garden of Eden in Mesopotamia, between the Tigris and Euphrates rivers. The Third Garden of Eden began on 15+ acres in Sedona, Arizona in the 1990s and relocated to 165 acres in Tumacácori, Arizona in 2007. The sacred gardens foster a protective and spiritual energy reflecting the souls and celestial personalities who live and work there, becoming a sacred drawing power and spiritual administrative center of the planet in the future.
Holy Spirit — the ministering spirit circuit of the Universe Mother Spirit that is one of three distinct spirit influences in the hearts and minds of mortals in aiding them to make higher and spiritized choices

J

Jerusem — the capital world of our administrative system of Satania

L

light and life — stages of planetary evolution, where consistently more and more stabilization of souls and the planet transpire into harmony and peace
local universe — an administrative grouping of planets and stars; ruled by a Creator Son and Creative Daughter; the local universe we live in is Nebadon

Lucifer — a celestial personality (Primary Lanonandek Son) who was the former System Sovereign of Satania. He rebelled against God, creating the Lucifer Manifesto of unbridled liberty, and leading countless personalities into rebellion with him.
Lucifer Rebellion — a spiritual rebellion led by Lucifer; began approximately 200,000 years ago and is now nearing an end via the adjudication by the Bright and Morning Star

M

Machiventa Melchizedek — a celestial personality of the order of Melchizedek Sons. He initially visited Urantia approximately 4,000 years ago, living in Salem (present site of Jerusalem) during the times of Abraham, who was Machiventa's pupil. He is the Melchizedek referred to in the Bible. Since December 1989, he has been serving as the Planetary Prince of Urantia, working in the spiritual administration of the planet in the fifth dimension and above.
Mandate of the Bright and Morning Star, the* — the God-given authority given to humans to take responsibility to be the world's spiritual leaders at this time in history; held by Gabriel of Urantia and Niánn Emerson Chase
mansion world(s) — planets in another dimension where souls go to upon death; the beginning of the after-life, where souls gain new morontia bodies and live on morontian worlds
morontia — the phase between the material and spiritual realms of the universe; semi-spiritual (part physical, part spiritual in nature/design)
morontia bodies — the 570 progressive, semi-spirit bodies a soul inhabits as he or she ascends after the mortal life and before becoming a pure spirit being
morontia counselor* — a trained psychospiritual counselor who provides morontia counseling
morontia counseling* — counseling that is concerned with the spiritual progression, fulfillment of destiny purpose, and personality actualization of an ascending son or daughter
morontia mota — higher levels of human and superhuman philosophy, incorporating principles and values of the highest moral standards and ethics
morontia temple — a huge and spectacular structure built on a planet for special ceremonies of the planet, including the transition phase of a mortal body being transformed into a beginning light body or morontia body upon Thought-Adjuster fusion, under the direction of Celestial Overcontrol
Mother-circuited* — representing the qualities of the Universe Mother Spirit, much like a human mother, in responses: gentle, soft, submissive, yielding, kind, giving, patient, etc.
Mystery Monitor — *See* Thought Adjuster

N

Nebadon — the name of our local universe, ruled by the Universe Father (Christ Michael) and His complement, the Universe Mother Spirit

O

Orvonton — the name of our superuniverse
ovan soul* — a soul who has lived before (on this world or another). On this planet ovan souls are either starseed or second-time Urantians.
Overcontrol* — *See* Celestial Overcontrol

P

physics of rebellion* — the actual physics and measurable, scientific study of the effects that rebellion against God and His divine pattern has on the bodies and souls of evolutionary mortals; a form of ascension science
Planetary Headquarters — *See* First Planetary Sacred Home
Planetary Prince — a celestial personality or on rare occasion a human responsible for ruling a planet spiritually; the spiritual leader of the world
point of origin* — the planet and local universe a mortal soul originated from during their very first life and existence on an evolutionary world. Most of the nearly seven billion souls on present-day Urantia have this planet Earth (in the local universe of Nebadon) as their point of origin. Approximately 500,000,000 souls on Urantia are starseed, with a point of origin in another universe.
point-of-origin reconstruction* — the process of a person who is in a fallen state returning to their more good and true states
psychic circle(s) — levels of personality development/attainment, based on stabilization of spiritual and mindal capacities, including manifesting the fruits of the Spirit

R

repersonalization* — when an existing soul is born as a baby in a new body on an evolutionary planet
revelatory religion — information given (revealed) by God and celestial personalities directly to mortals. Revelatory religion contrasts evolutionary religions, which contain both some truths and falsehoods.

S

Salvington — the name of the capital world of our local universe (Nebadon), where Christ Michael lives and reigns
Satania — the name of our administrative system, currently ruled by Lanaforge, our System Sovereign.
second-time Urantian* — a soul who lived one life previously on Earth (Urantia)
Son-circuited* — representing the qualities of the balance between the Universe Father and Mother with strong human father traits and gentle human mother qualities in responses. *See also* Father-circuited and Mother-circuited.
Spirit of Truth — the spirit of Christ Michael within you, given to help mortals discern truth in their lives
starseed* — soul whose point of origin is another planet/universe and has lived at least one other life not on Urantia
superuniverse — an administrative distinction of local universes grouped together, consisting of 100,000 universes when finally complete
system — an administrative distinction of planets grouped together, consisting of 1,000 inhabited worlds when finally complete

T

third dimension* — the present dominant culture on Urantia; the "mainstream"; the lower, fallen system of the mass-consciousness
Thought Adjuster — a fragment of God, the Universal Father, that lives within you and attempts to adjust your thoughts toward God and more spiritual things
Threefold Spirit — the combined spirit circuitry connection between mortals and the Universal Father (via the Thought Adjuster), the local universe Creator Son (via the Spirit of Truth), and the Universe Mother Spirit (via the Holy Spirit)
tron therapy* — a special touch therapy coordinating with celestial forces, used in healing of the body, mind, and soul

U

union of souls* — a group of like-minded souls seeking God's will and attempting to manifest it; this union creates a special form of measurable energy
Universal Father — God, the First Source and Center, the Father of all creation and creatures
Universe Father — the Creator Son of a local universe. In our universe of Nebadon, the Universe Father is Jesus Christ Michael**.** *See also* Creator Son.
Universe Mother Spirit — a Creative Daughter, celestial personality who co-rules a local universe with a Creator Son/Universe Father as complements to each other
Urantia — cosmic name for our planet, "Earth"

Urantian Reservist* — Urantian human mortals assigned and trained to aid in times of planetary emergency, particularly spiritual crises; a.k.a. change agents

Urantians* — individuals whose point of origin is on this earth, Urantia. Urantians are younger souls with no past-life experiences. Most people on the planet are Urantians. *See also* First-time Urantian and Second-time Urantian.

About the Authors

Gabriel of Urantia & Niánn Emerson Chase

Gabriel of Urantia and Niánn Emerson Chase are spiritual leaders, pastors, teachers, counselors, authors, and motivational speakers. They founded Global Community Communications Alliance in 1989 (located in Arizona, USA, with approximately 100 members), and together they are the human spiritual leaders and administrators of Divine Administration there. They founded the Soulistic Medical Institute and Soulistic Hospice, also in Arizona. Additionally they serve as the Executive Directors of the Alternative Voice, an international periodical, produced by Global Community Communications Alliance, which fuses spirituality with activism.

Both Gabriel of Urantia and Niánn Emerson Chase have been proactive in the spiritual, social, and environmental arenas for decades, standing up for justice and godly choices. Together they hold the Mandate of the Bright and Morning Star, a spiritual mandate focused on creating global change to assist our planet shifting into higher levels of consciousness and responsibility for each other and the world. Their Global Change Teachings present very real solutions to bring about global change through spiritual unity, without uniformity.

Gabriel of Urantia and Niánn Emerson Chase also established and direct Avalon Organic Gardens, Farm, and Ranch, 165-acres located along the beautiful Santa Cruz River in Tumacácori, Arizona. The gardens provide year-round educational gardening tours and workshops and host a variety of seasonal events, including annually an Easter Celebration, World Peace and Prayer Day, Interdependence Day, a Celebration of Education, Earth Sustainability Day, and an Autumn Harvest Festival.

Gabriel of Urantia

Gabriel of Urantia, originally from Pittsburgh, Pennsylvania, has authored several books, including the first two volumes of *The Cosmic Family* as well as his autobiography, *The Divine New Order, Into the New Millennium*. *The Cosmic Family* volumes are fundamental as a basis for understanding the current state of our planet and how to truly begin creating global change on both individual and corporate levels.

Gabriel of Urantia is also an accomplished musician, songwriter/singer, and performer. In 1985, he pioneered the first New Age "Vocal" album, *Unicorn Love*. Now he has introduced another unique style of music, CosmoPop®, to the world, performing major outdoor concerts nationwide. As of the publishing of this book, Gabriel of Urantia has produced five CDs and is often in the recording studio working on future albums and projects. He has an award-winning concert DVD (which won an Aurora Award Gold Award for "Musical Live Concert") featuring his accomplished nine-piece band, The Bright & Morning Star Band.

Niánn Emerson Chase

Niánn Emerson Chase grew up on four different Native American reservations in Arizona and, after earning her degree, returned to the San Carlos Apache Reservation where she lived and taught for fifteen years. Since her early childhood, with an explorer's nature inherent in her ancestors Meriwether Lewis and Ralph Waldo Emerson, Niánn has had an unquenchable thirst for knowledge and the character of one who truly loves discovery and the adventure of life. Her life's experiences, growing up with native people, roaming the desert lands of the Southwest, and pursuing her search to know God in a higher way are shared in her writings. Her articles have been published in various periodicals including: *New Thought Journal, Connecting Link, Communities*

Magazine, *Quantum Thoughts,* and *Inner Words* and as the leading writer for Global Community Communications Alliance's *Alternative Voice*.

Niánn Emerson Chase is the Director of the Global Community Communications Schools, higher spiritual-based schools for adults, teens, and children. She also coordinates Global Community Communications Publishing's endeavors and is the head of the editing team for all book production.

Global Community Communications Alliance and Divine Administration

Global Community Communications Alliance is a church supporting: a religious order and EcoVillage of 100+ international members living in community (with thousands of local and international supporters and readers); Avalon Organic Gardens, Farm, and Ranch; Personality Integration Rehabilitation Program for Teens and Adults; Global Family Legal Services. In addition, Global Community Communications Alliance's affiliates and supporting nonprofit organizations Soulistic Medical Institute and Soulistic Hospice, and Global Change Multi-Media also support ministry programs.

Founded in 1989 by Gabriel of Urantia (www.GabrielOfUrantia.info, www.GabrielOfUrantia.net, www.GabrielOfUrantia.com) and Niánn Emerson Chase, Global Community Communications Alliance is located in southern Arizona in the charming, historic southwest towns of Tubac and Tumacácori—a sacred area known as "the Palm of God's Hand."

Find out more about our many local and global church programs, services, and related humanitarian efforts listed here:

World-Wide Sunday ServicesSM
Open to the public and webcast via Internet.
(520) 603-9932

Avalon Organic Gardens, Farm, & RanchSM
165-acre farm and ranch in southern Arizona, using spiritually-based principles and permaculture practices.
Also a Community Supported Agriculture (CSA) provider.
www.AvalonGardens.org • (520) 603-9932

Soulistic Medical Institute & Soulistic Hospice
Offers healthcare by professionals whose expertise involves various healing modalities that encompass the soul, mind, and body.
www.SoulisticMedicalInstitute.org • (520) 398-3970
Hospice (520) 398-2333

Personality Integration Rehabilitation Program℠ for Teens and Adults

Assisting those socially-disappointed souls in their psychospiritual healing process.
www.pirp.info • (520) 603-9932

Friendly Hands Vocational Training

Spiritual Training Apprenticeship Programs in a wide range of career fields.
www.FriendlyHandsVocational.org • (520) 603-9932

Global Family Legal Services

Legal aid in various fields focusing on immigration for low-income individuals and families in need.
www.GlobalFamilyLegalServices.org • (928) 282-2590

Global Community Communications Publishing™

Publishing continuing epochal revelation and related materials as well as Global Change Teachings and other spiritually-oriented texts.
www.GlobalCommunityCommunicationsPublishing.org
(520) 603-9932

***Alternative Voice*™**

Quarterly periodical that addresses the many crises of our world, fusing spirituality with activism.
www.AlternativeVoice.org • (520) 603-9932

Spirit Steps Tours℠

Offering enlightening tours for the seeking sojourner and eco-tourist.
www.SpiritSteps.org • (520) 398-2655

Global Community Communications Schools℠

Incorporating the highest truths from many world religions as well as continuing epochal revelation.
www.GlobalCommunityCommunicationsSchools.org
(520) 603-9932

Out of the Way Galleria℠

An eclectic blend of created art contributed by local artisans and donors.
www.OutOfTheWayGalleria.org • (520) 398-9409

CosmoArt Studio℠
Blending the talents of many artists in creating spiritually-inspiring art through humility and cooperation.
www.CosmoArt.org • (520) 603-9932

Planetary Family Services℠
Provides services to create, embellish, and bring Godly energy to your home environment.
www.PlanetaryFamilyServices.org • (520) 668-7786

Global Change Multi-Media
www.GlobalChangeMultiMedia.org • (520) 398-2542
www.GlobalChangeTools.org

Divisions of Global Change Multi-Media:

Future Studios℠
Recording studio and live-entertainment venue, presenting performers from around the world in a dynamic and positive environment, free from smoke, alcohol, and drugs. Events can be viewed live on-line through World-Wide Webcasts.
Moving soon to southern Arizona, Tucson area
www.FutureStudios.org • (520) 398-2542

Global Change Music℠
Nonprofit record label offers musicians recording opportunities using professional world-class equipment for voice and instrumental training.
www.GlobalChangeMusic.org • (520) 398-2542

The Musicians That Need To Be Heard Network℠
Provides opportunities for musicians to communicate their music messages without spiritual compromise.
www.MusiciansThatNeedToBeHeardNetwork.org
(520) 398-2542

Global Change Radio℠
Internet radio station broadcasting live and on-demand audio webcasts, including talk radio on various religious and social themes.
www.GlobalChangeRadio.org • (520) 398-2542

Global Change TelevisionSM

Internet television station offering live webcasts worldwide with a variety of programs of spiritual content, on demand.
www.GlobalChangeTelevision.org • (520) 398-2542

Global Change FilmsSM

Presenting educational, mind-expanding, and thought-provoking films that strive to raise the consciousness of the planet. Soon Global Change Films will produce major motion pictures with a spiritual emphasis.
www.GlobalChangeFilms.org • (520) 398-2542

Future Studios CinemaSM

Working with filmmakers and distributors of independent, pro-activist, and educational films and documentaries which motivate spiritually thought-provoking group dialogue for the public at Future Studios.
www.FutureStudiosCinema.org • (520) 398-2542

Global Change Theater CompanySM

Dedicated to writing, performing, and staging plays and various higher-consciousness, inspirational, dramatic productions where students receive training and opportunities to participate in theatrical shows and workshops.
(520) 398-2542

Global Change Multi-Media Distribution CompanySM

Distributes music, DVDs, books, magazines, and any product that would be considered by its parent company to be a Global Change Tool for the dissemination of revelation and spiritually-uplifting information through media materials.

Global Change Multi-Media ProductionsSM

Professional audio, video, and Internet service producing spiritual and educational message media, via Internet video streaming, live webcasting, graphic design, and CD and video/DVD media production.
(520) 398-2542

Global Community Communications Alliance

P.O. Box 4910, Tubac, AZ 85646 USA • (520) 603-9932

info@GlobalCommunityCommunicationsAlliance.org
www.GlobalCommunityCommunicationsAlliance.org

Soulistic Medical Institute

Healing Soul, Mind, and Body

In order for the body to truly heal, the soul must heal. At the Soulistic Medical Institute we understand the key role each patient plays in his or her own healing process and the importance of a wholehearted desire to *heal holistically*, rather than just finding a more immediate "cure" for what ails an individual.

With this philosophy in mind, the members of the healing team at the Soulistic Medical Institute are trained to discern the root cause of illness—whether physical, emotional, or spiritual. They work as a *team* of professionals, for they understand the interdependence of the various body systems and the related interdependent treatment methods that may be needed. At the time of the publication of this book, the healing team consists of a physician, clinical psychologist, registered nurses, and massage therapists, all licensed in the state of Arizona, as well as Reiki practitioners at a master's level. Personal transmissions are available when appropriate by Gabriel of Urantia. All primary staff practitioners are religious order workers of Global Community Communications Alliance who volunteer their talents to serve humanity. A sliding-scale plan is available to better serve all people of various economic levels.

At the Soulistic Medical Institute, a healing plan for each unique soul is designed and implemented with you to meet your healing needs and circumstances, based on the teachings in this book as well as even more advanced teachings. This may include morontia counseling (a form of psychospiritual counseling), conventional and alternative medicine, and tron therapy (one of the highest forms of touch healing available on the planet today). Additionally, the incorporation of herbal and nutritional advice, and/or massage and exercise planning may be recommended parts of an individual's healing program. Residency programs are available.

This approach to healing is both very old and brand new, in that it brings full circle every soul's calling to meet his or her God-given destiny and to share his or her health and blessings in such a way that all may have life and have it more abundantly. The Soulistic Medical Institute understands what Gabriel of Urantia teaches: "The secret of the mystery of illness and healing has to do with meeting one's destiny and following God's perfect will to do that."

The Soulistic Medical Institute endeavors to serve all people of all economic levels who have a sincere desire to actively participate in their own healing process.

If the teachings in this book resonate with you and you feel this approach to healing would benefit you or someone you love, please contact the Soulistic Medical Institute to find out more about our services.

If you are a healing practitioner who resonates with our philosophies, please contact the Soulistic Medical Institute for more information in exploring the possibilities of joining our healing team as part of our auxiliary staff.

Soulistic Medical Institute and **Soulistic Hospice**
a nonprofit organization

Your financial donations help us to serve more individuals with financial hardships.

P.O. Box 1990, Tubac, AZ 85646-1990 USA
(520) 398-3970 • (520) 398-2333 Hospice
info@soulisticmedicalinstitute.org
www.soulisticmedicalinstitute.org

Other Titles
by Gabriel of Urantia and Niánn Emerson Chase
available from
Global Community Communications Publishing

The Divine New Order
by Gabriel of Urantia
Autobiography of Gabriel of Urantia and the history
of the beginnings of Global Community Communications Alliance

The Cosmic Family, Volume I
as transmitted through Gabriel of Urantia
Continuing Fifth Epochal Revelation,
Papers 197-228 succeeding *The URANTIA Book*

Messages to Urantia, 1997-2000
as transmitted through Gabriel of Urantia
A collection of 19 sacred messages
from celestial beings addressing the state of our world, Urantia

Global Change Teachings for the New Millennium,
Series One, Two, & Three
by Gabriel of Urantia and Niánn Emerson Chase
Teachings to assist the planet's transition
into the first stage of light and life

The Best of the Film Industry—Movies You Don't Want to Miss!
compiled by Gabriel of Urantia
A list of films that educate, challenge, and expand the consciousness

Making the Most of Media Exposure for Global Change
Versus Our Experience with the Media
by Gabriel of Urantia and Niánn Emerson Chase
Firsthand account of experiences with corporate-controlled media

Spiritual Quotes
by Gabriel of Urantia
A collection of spiritual insights and wisdom addressing
many of life's facets

Breinigsville, PA USA
03 August 2010
242951BV00003B/4/P

9 780982 242308